Corona Time

Philosophy of Action Design and Multiplicity

Book 9

Dan Paul

Chapter 1

Vanished

The population vanished overnight. Could a war do that? No, not so fast. The streets were empty as far as the eye could see. Finally, people got a break from the endless work and dreadful commuting, a break they hadn't had for many years. The moratorium allowed workers an extended vacation. Many hated the commute, the dangerous, polluted freeways, horrendous accidents, and the endless struggle of work. In boring jobs, it was hard to stop wondering why she was working so hard to make things people didn't need. Most of it would end up in the garbage. Why make more stuff when it only speeds up the momentum to extinction?

Some people get the virus, and some don't.

Who will get the virus? In the beginning, it needed to be clarified. The government was caught off guard and was unwilling to admit that there was a problem and that something should be done about it. The pro-Trump and conservative media echoed the lies of the president. Other media was critical and informative, but the call to action did not come from the government. It came from those who suffered and died from the virus, those who had to live with the consequences of the failure of the government. The idea of wearing a mask was utterly foreign, except for people from areas that had worn masks before. You'd see a few on the streets or in the subway. They knew how to do it. No one had to explain why they had to wear a mask. They had experience and didn't question public health, an uncommon idea to most. Quickly, the virus spread in New York City and rapidly showed its force.

Conditions of the virus

The conditions of the virus's host, the human body, determine how the virus will interact with a human. What are the conditions? What is the age of a person? Younger people are less vulnerable. The most susceptible are people above the age of 65. What is the condition of the immune system? If the immune system is not functioning well or has to fight heart disease, cancer, or an auto-immune disease, the virus is more likely to subdue the human. What is the body mass index of the person? Are they overweight or obese? The more overweight they are, the more likely they will have significant problems with the virus. What is the temperature of the environment where the host lives? If the temperature is consistently above 70 degrees Fahrenheit, the virus is less likely to spread than if the temperature is consistently below 60 degrees Fahrenheit. Under the right conditions, the virus can multiply.

Older people are more likely to get the virus.

As time passed, it became more obvious who would have big problems with the virus. People above 60 had the most chance of a severe illness. Anyone with a weak heart, lungs, liver, brain, or sickness would be more likely to die from the virus. A friend of mine got the virus. He was overweight with heart issues, but he could still walk and function before he got the virus. The virus nearly killed him. He wanted to go to the hospital, but they turned him down. Perhaps that's what saved his life. He said he was close to dying more than once and that the virus was the biggest fight that he had ever fought. At times, he didn't think he would make it. Eventually, he hit the worst and gradually improved, but that took a long time. He said the doctors told him that because he had gotten the virus so severely, he probably wouldn't have to worry about it again because his immune system had become empowered.

Nursing homes

Nursing homes provide services for older adults who can't live independently and have no one to care for them. Often, conditions for living in a nursing home may not be so good. The staff may be limited. The facilities may need fresh air or air filters, which must be properly cleaned. Nursing home patients often have compromised immune systems, circulation systems, nervous systems, and other sicknesses. These are the perfect conditions for the virus to spread and become lethal.

Pernicious virus

One of the most terrifying aspects of the virus is that it can spread very quickly without anyone becoming aware of it. Many people can have the virus and not have any symptoms. In that case, people feel fine and may spread the virus far and wide, including to the people they love the most and people who are most likely to die if they get the virus. To prevent this from happening, the government instructed people to remain inside as much as possible. If you must go out, wear a mask and avoid getting closer than 6 feet from another person. If you get symptoms, you must take a test to verify that it's the Coronavirus. If you have the virus, you must stay away from anyone else until you test negative. It was as if the body of the social world became paralyzed.

Strategy to avoid dying from the virus

Eventually, the way to avoid the virus was to carefully follow the social distancing guidelines until a vaccine is available. When the vaccine is ready, take the vaccine, and hopefully, it will work. People wore masks, stayed 3-6 feet away from each other, and quarantined if they were exposed to people who had the virus. After the governor shut down the state of New York in March 2020, most businesses, museums, or parks had few people, which reduced your chances of getting the virus. Some people quarantined as much as they could. Some didn't leave their home for months. Some people wore two masks at once.

When will the vaccine be available?

Typical estimates of the time it takes to make and test a potential vaccine are over a few years. With the virus killing hundreds and sometimes thousands of people a day, the pressure to reduce that time was high, but how could it be done safely? If the vaccine had one flaw, many people could die or suffer tremendous pain. If that was the case, would they admit the problem and do something about it? Eventually, the vaccine came out. Most people didn't get severe side effects. In general, the vaccines were tolerated. By 2024, most people have had the vaccine or the virus and now have some immunity. If people get the virus, they will have more immunity and are more likely to survive.

Which vaccine to take?

Nearly every week after April 2020, a company announced that it would make a vaccine to save the world from the virus. Should we take the first one that comes out or wait for something better? How would the government make sure the vaccine is safe? Can we trust the government? These and other questions consumed our intellects.

Was this a disease where the rules don't apply? If you take care of yourself, will you have a better chance? Will everyone who gets it die? Will the vaccine work without question? Will the virus mutate like the flu and other similar viruses? The ideas kept zooming around.

Government preparation

Starting with George W. Bush, the federal government made plans to prepare the country for a pandemic. The government set up the appropriate response if a pandemic happened. The public would have to be educated, and businesses and government would have to change how they did their work.

People would have to wear masks, and indoor events with more than a few people would have to be limited or canceled. Widespread testing would have to be available for free. Restrictions on the density of people indoors would have to be enforced. People would have to stop doing what they had been doing and adapt to the virus.

I learned about it from Red; he told me they were indefinitely closing the restaurant. The government shut it down. There was nothing anyone could do about it. They had to lock up and stop operating. We talked about the logic of the shutdown. If the virus spread too fast and made too many people sick at once, the hospitals would be overwhelmed and unable to care for everyone. This could lead to the collapse of hospitals. So we washed hands, sprayed disinfectant on the hallways, doorknobs, handrails, mailboxes, and outside handrails, and disinfected the public halls using diluted bleach water. We wore masks as directed and boosted our nutrition with vitamin D3, greens, herbs, protein, and bone broth.

Contradictions

We accept heart disease and cancer. Combined, they cause over 1 million deaths per year. Many of these deaths are preventable. We don't shut down the economy to stop it. Cigarettes, internal combustion vehicles, alcohol, and meat cause heart disease and cancer, are legal and pushed on the public 24 hours a day, seven days a week, and we don't stop it. The big reason for shutting down the economy was to prevent a collapse of the medical system and a surge of casualties. Was it a risky decision? Indeed, people disagreed on what to do. Some states shut down the economy, and some didn't. Shutting down the economy caused many people to lose their jobs. The government pumped money into the economy to help those in need. The US lost a large number of people during the pandemic. Many of those were older people with health problems.

Chapter 2

Family Responses

Like others, families were stressed by the challenges of the pandemic. If one person brings the virus through the door, everyone else will likely get it. Typically, the virus had the least impact on children and the most on older people. Families with members over 60 had the most to be concerned about, especially if they had an existing condition, if they could easily get infected, or if they were short on caregivers. In many families, the parents worked from home, and the children used the Internet for school activities. This added more pressure to the household. If the Internet broke, the pressure would rise enormously. Families in small apartments or tiny houses would have to share the same room while each person is working or going to school. For families that lost income, the strain was even more significant. It was uncertain what would happen after the pandemic. People didn't know what would happen to the economy or if the vaccine would work.

Families with Covid

For families with the virus, going to the hospital could be a death sentence. Hospitals lacked nurses, doctors, beds, ventilators, equipment, and supplies. Even worse was that they had no cure. If one person got the virus at home, they all would likely get it. People over 60 with compromised circulatory, respiratory, or immune system problems were likely to have serious complications that may result in death. Some families had more than one death from the virus. At the beginning of the pandemic, hospital workers were overwhelmed and couldn't get the supplies and equipment needed to fight the virus. In that emergency, they couldn't let family members in the hospital see their loved ones. Now, if someone dies, the family would have to arrange for services to bury or cremate the person. All of this led to enormous amounts of pain, stress, and agony.

Pressure in isolation

The pandemic exploded at the beginning of 2020 in New York City. The government shut down the economy in March 2020. Eventually, companies were able to set up people to work from home. Schools also had to adjust and set up students to take classes from home. With more than one person using the Internet for work, school, and other activities, internet services may be stretched to the limit. Service may be compromised if everyone in the area is on the Internet. Some rooms had better service than others. This puts pressure on people to work in the same room, which could mean two or more people listening and speaking simultaneously. As the chaos increased, the potential for stress and conflict rose. Remember that people were supposed to leave their housing only if necessary. This meant that people had to work and go to school in the same room and couldn't leave the house or apartment, almost like solitary confinement. No one could go out to dinner, see a movie, or attend a theater event. You could go out for a walk, but you had to wear masks and keep 6 feet away from anyone you did not live with.

Families with no Internet service

Some families did not have Internet service. If they had children and had to go to school, some schools would set up computers so that the children could take classes on the computers at school. They had to wear masks, and the desks and computers had to be 6 feet apart. The experience was bizarre and alienating. At a time when students needed social interaction, connection, and friends the most, they had to come to school and isolate themselves from the people they wanted the most: fellow students and teachers.

Depression and Mental Illness

The virus spreads death and illness across the world. The second wave of all that pain reverberated through the hearts and minds of people everywhere. Anxiety and depression swept over families that caught the virus. First, people had to take care of the sick. Someone could have no symptoms, have mild symptoms, or much worse. If you were over 60, were obese, and had an existing condition, the chances of getting very sick and dying were much higher than the rest of the population. Combining an unknown economic future and whether or not a family member will survive the pandemic made anxiety and depression spread like wildfire. In a big way, the pandemic challenged the ability of families to adapt.

Friendships and High School

The social isolation of the pandemic made it impossible for children to interact with friends. If the child was entering a new school, they didn't have the chance to establish friends in the new school. This generated a lot of problems for kids who were already stressed from the pressure to get good grades, get to school on time, and negotiate time with friends, teachers, and family. Large numbers of children found it quite challenging to focus on schoolwork. Parents working from home, people sick and dying from the virus, and tension from family members who lived with each other 24 hours a day, seven days a week generated the conditions for students to fall into anxiety, depression, and hopelessness. For the fortunate, therapy provided a way to cope with the pandemic.

Coping with mental health

Some children had been going to therapy, which could be an advantage. Other children were pressured to go, especiallyif they talked about hurting themselves or others. Online meetings, which were new to most, also provided a way to beat back the omniscient threat of isolation, loneliness, anxiety, and depression. People were allowed to go outside if they wore masks and stayed 6 feet apart. Playing outside was a lower-risk activity. Some people took chances and let their children play outside with other children. It spelled hope for children stuck inside even if it was one other friend. School counselors, therapists, zoom meetings, and parents gathered forces to minimize the impact of the virus.

Financial Impact

Non-essential businesses, including bars, restaurants, and hotels, needed more work and had to lay off large numbers of people. Some had yet to learn where the money would come from to pay the bills. During the first three months of the pandemic, unemployment rose rapidly to one of the highest levels ever. While the government did provide money during the pandemic, some families did not receive any money. Non-white and low-income white families had to struggle to afford to live.

Non-family households during the pandemic.

If you lived alone and could avoid the virus, you could make it through without huge problems, but many who lived alone faced severe issues even if they didn't get the virus. Most social gatherings that included more than a few people were canceled. Social isolation during the pandemic increased anxiety and depression. Without a friend or family member, how could they release their pain by talking face-to-face with someone?

Families with members who died from the virus.

The virus walloped some families. If the members were older and had significant health problems like heart disease, obesity, or poor circulation, two or more family members could die from the virus. If a family member remains, they may or may not be able to arrange for a funeral. Depending on the funeral, friends and relatives would need to be notified. People gather to share emotions, support, and memories. The gathering may be a simple spreading of the ashes, formal burial, and often with lunch. If no one remains and no family members are alive, the state may arrange a way to bury or cremate the deceased.

The financial impact of losing a family member who provides income, food, and shelter can be devastating. Some have family, friends, and government that can help. Others may be in dire straights and depend on what hospice can offer.

Chapter 3

Who gets the virus?

The government was caught off guard when the virus attacked. Like invisible smoke, it spread far and wide. They had no idea what to do or how to do it. Leadership was vacant, watching TV, playing golf, and eating junk food. Most Republicans believe that people should get health insurance and care for themselves. The government should not be helping people stay healthy. The role of the government is to help people get money so they can pay for health insurance. So, Trump dismantled the government infrastructure and personnel to respond to the virus. The slow response of the government meant that 1 million people would die from the virus, and many others would have to suffer needlessly because the government did not take action. So, the government realized who would get the virus. They knew it was happening and did little to stop it. People living with others in confined areas were more likely to get the virus. Those include frontline workers in hospitals, grocery store workers, and people in homeless shelters, prisons, and nursing homes. So, who would get the virus?

The following people were most vulnerable to the virus.

People in contact with people coming from other countries with the virus.

People with weakened immune systems.

People who did not wear a mask or avoid crowds, especially indoors.

People who use transit without a mask.

People with heart disease, autoimmune disease, lung problems, circulation problems, and obese people.

The virus attacks weak people.

This can include people with a lousy diet who don't eat foods that are good for the immune system. Diets with many highly processed foods include candy bars, diet sodas, and enriched white bread—foods with many ingredients that include bromides, stabilizers, and dyes. Your body may not function if your diet consists of many fast food items like hamburgers, chicken nuggets, and fried foods. Weakness may come from stress.

People loaded with stress may have problems with the virus.

Some people work more than one job. Performing well at two or more jobs per day may take time. Problems getting to and from work may include:

•Breathing pollution.

•Stress from driving a vehicle.

•Stress from being late to work.

If family members or friends are sick, they may be unable to get food, water, or medicine. Some need help getting to the emergency room, making an appointment, or attending a permitted gathering. Most people with less income have more worries about how to pay for housing, insurance, transportation, and food. Stress makes people feel tired and overwhelmed. Sometimes, this increases arguments and conflict as people cannot function.

Where could people go?

If you are not sick and don't know anyone else who is ill, you may not feel compelled to take precautions. When the first surge of the virus came to New York City, people were not supposed to leave home. There were no tests at that time, so it was difficult to know if you had the virus or a cold or flu. You could have all the symptoms of the Coronavirus and not have the Coronavirus. People could go most places if they wore a mask stayed 6 feet apart, and were outside.

Frontline Workers

People who worked with people with the virus were more likely to get the virus. People who drove ambulances and worked in emergency rooms and hospitals had a much higher chance of getting the virus. Initially, there were not enough masks and protective equipment for emergency frontline workers to reduce the spread of the virus. Some frontline workers slept in their cars to avoid infecting their families. The most important people to protect were not getting the help they needed. If you worked in an occupation that had to operate during the pandemic, you were more likely to get the virus. Groceries stores, gas stations, hardware stores, and building supply stores had to stay open during the pandemic. If transit was operating, the transit workers, including bus drivers and train conductors, were exposed to more people who may have the virus.

People in Nursing Homes were quite vulnerable.

Nursing homes are places for people who can't live at home. Most are older adults with health problems. Workers in nursing homes often go from patient to patient and may spread the virus. Sometimes, these buildings aren't well-ventilated, which may help spread the virus. Many patients died in nursing homes. With hospitals at capacity, where could they go?

Homeless Shelters

People in homeless shelters were more likely to get the virus. With fewer chances to social distance, wash hands, and avoid other people, the chances of touching surfaces with the virus, getting sneezed on, or making physical contact with somebody who had the virus were high. Up-to-date information was yet to be available. When the virus started, masks and gloves were in short supply, and people didn't have money and probably could not afford it.

Prisons

Prisons contain many people in a confined area. Priority was given to protective equipment for hospital workers, then frontline workers, and the last priority was to give it to prisoners. Access to soap and water for handwashing may have been limited. One photo of prisoners from El Salvador shows 20 to 50 prisoners with no clothes on except for a simple towel, sitting immediately next to other prisoners. They had their arms around the other prisoners and were so close that it was pretty likely that many would get and spread the virus.

People who contact many during the day are most likely to get the virus. Since people can have the virus without symptoms, knowing who had the virus was impossible, especially before the testing kits were available. That's the most insidious time of the virus. There was a lot of uncertainty at the time.

Meatpacking workers

Meatpacking plants were ideal conditions for the virus to spread. Workers labor close to each other in moist and cool conditions, and some plants employ underage workers. Plants were forced to close after workers tested positive for the virus. After closing down, cleaning up, and adapting protocols, workers had less chance of getting the virus.

Chapter 4

Keeping healthy in Corona time

Frontline workers

Healthcare workers were on the front lines of the pandemic. Large numbers of sick people overwhelmed nurses, doctors, and support staff. Medical supplies to prevent the spread of the virus, such as masks, gloves, and sanitation supplies, were in short supply. Healthcare workers were critical to everyone's health and security, and now they were in jeopardy; they had to make up for inaction and incompetence from the federal government. For these workers, it was nearly impossible to stay healthy. They had to work long hours without equipment and a viable solution to help people stay alive during the pandemic. Some slept in their cars or away from home to prevent the spread of the virus to other family members. Tragically, nurses and doctors got sick and died helping others fight the virus.

1918 Pandemic

Most Americans have little experience with a pandemic. The last major pandemic was in 1918-1920. They could only stop it once they ended social gatherings, stopped attending schools, and implemented social distancing requirements. Other methods include the following:

Staying home.

Wash hands frequently and vigorously.

avoiding public gatherings

using masks and gloves

avoid touching items outside the house

no sneezing or spitting in public

shut down businesses and government offices

Eventually, the most vulnerable people died. Another group got the virus and grew immune to the virus. Some people living in isolation were never exposed to the virus. Some estimates say 50 million people died during the pandemic of 1918.

Can I get the virus when I get food at the store?

For many, the best option to stay healthy was to isolate yourself from everyone else. People stayed in their homes but needed food supplies and equipment. When going to the store, it was essential to wear a mask and to wear gloves. It was initially unclear how the virus was spreading. Could I touch anything in the store and transfer the virus from my hands or gloves to my face or close enough to get the virus? Also, how long would the virus be contagious? Going to the store was one of the more risky behaviors. Without vigilance, it's easy to repeat habits. I usually touch the door, counters, food, boxes, and money. Could I get it from the cashier? It's easy to forget the new rules in a place that has always been safe.

Spraying diluted bleach water

I was living in a six-floor walk-up building at the time. I wanted to do something to make our building as safe as possible. Typically, I would never use bleach, but when I did some research, it seemed like it could be used with minimal risk. I found a bottle and some bleach. I mixed a teaspoon of bleach per gallon of water. Then, every day or so, I would go from the sixth floor down, through the public halls and stairways to the outside. I would start spraying the door knobs of each apartment, then the handrails, post office boxes, outside door, railings, and the handles for opening the garbage containers. Since it was easy to spray quickly, I also did the entrance to the basement. I tried to do it when no one was around. I wore a mask and would spray in the air if I thought the virus was floating. Did it work? Using the least energy and money was a preventative measure.

The main strategy.

So, what's the big idea about staying healthy? What is the primary strategy? If we prevented the virus from entering our apartment until a vaccine was ready, we could avoid suffering from the most intense response to the virus. Once we get the vaccine, we can develop the immunity required to minimize the impact of the virus. As long as we didn't get sick until the vaccine was ready, we could avoid the worst impacts of the virus.

Fundamentals

The following is a list of ways to avoid the virus and stay healthy:

Wear a mask and gloves as much as possible.

Stay 6 feet away from people.

Avoid indoor gatherings of people.

Avoid transit; walk and bicycle instead.

Gargle with mouthwash, especially after close encounters with the virus.

Take Vitamin D.

Shop when no one is in the store.

We were told to wash our hands frequently and be careful when touching door handles, faucet handles, handrails, and public infrastructure with hand use. It wasn't clear how the virus was spreading. One idea was that droplets from sneezing spread to surfaces, and that's how it spread. Another idea was that it spread like smoke, which is very light and could move far from the source. That's why a mask could protect you. If someone sneezed, who was close to you, at least you would have a layer of materials between you and the droplets. It could still spread. That's why people wore gloves and masks in the beginning. Gloves help prevent the spread. However, how it spreads still needs to be clarified. It was clear that it could spread very quickly, especially among large numbers of people congregating closely.

Chinese Response

In China, the government provides healthcare. Healthcare is not a commodity for sale to the highest bidder. The government is interested in minimizing the pain, suffering, and accidents that cause health problems because, ultimately, the government will have to pay. So, the Chinese shut down the economy. They took the most radical, direct action to eradicate the virus. They shut down a city of 10 million overnight, which was unthinkable in the West. In ten days, they tested everyone—another unlikely achievement in the US. So, if you wanted to stay healthy in China, you followed the orders of the government. You stayed inside, wore masks, and followed instructions. The Chinese government protected its people from the virus. Some videos show how the government roughed up some people to get them to comply. Is it better to do that or let people die from the virus?

Anti-mask and anti-vaccination ideas killed people.

The endless torrent of double and triple speak from the anti-mask and anti-vaccination populations led many people to endure enormous hardship and to their graves. Generally, the more Republican or against any change of the status quo, the more likely you would be to get and die from the virus. If you didn't wear a mask, wash your hands, or avoid large numbers of people gathered indoors, you were more likely to get the virus. Nearly every week, you would see another story about an anti-vax person on their deathbed denying that the virus is a problem or that they should have taken the vaccine.

People who denied that the virus was a problem died from the virus.

It was more than a bit ironic when liberals promoted ideas that would save the lives of their adversaries. Over and over, it would happen. People said the virus was a hoax and died from it. Others were less dogmatic and more pragmatic. With more to lose by ignoring the public health mandates, they complied with mandates to minimize the spread of the virus. Wearing a mask, washing hands, and avoiding groups larger than ten people were relatively easy to comply with. The ideas in the public mind shaped how people responded or didn't respond to the virus. In the US, freedom of speech was sending people to their graves in huge numbers.

MRNA virus

The Coronavirus is a Ribonucleic Acid (RNA) virus. It mutates quickly. Does that mean the vaccine would not be effective against virus variations? If you had the vaccine or the virus and were still alive, it's likely that a variation of the virus would not make you extremely sick. RNA is similar to the flu. There's a different strain of the virus every year. The immunity you've acquired from other flu viruses may or may not protect you from the yearly variations. When they make a vaccine against the current variation of the flu virus, it may or may not work. So, it's possible to take the vaccine and the booster shots and maintain enough immunity.

Chapter 5

You can't avoid the virus, so get it and be done with it

We looked for strategies to counter the virus at the beginning of the pandemic. It wasn't clear who was most vulnerable at the time, but ideas were floating around. People over 60 with a compromised circulatory, respiratory, or immune system were most likely to have more problems with the virus. Healthy people under 60 could get through it without significant issues. So, for a healthy person under 60, the question may arise, "Why not get the virus and be done with it?" I would have the antibodies to improve my immune system and wouldn't have to think about getting it again. At the time, it wasn't clear. If I get the virus, can I get it again? If I get the virus, how bad will it be? Will it be like the flu, or maybe I won't have any symptoms?

Avoid the virus with good hygiene.

We could avoid the virus. We did what the government said. We washed hands, wore masks, and kept a safe distance from other people. Also, I began spraying diluted bleach water on public hall railings, door knobs, mailboxes, and trash containers. We were cautious when we went shopping in the grocery stores and pharmacies. Was someone else in the building spreading the virus? One person told us they had been exposed to someone who tested positive. Months and months went by, and all of us kept testing negative. Some of the measures had worked, but how would we know?

Avoid the virus by leaving town.

The solution was obvious for people who had a house in the country, especially if they could work from home. Just move out. There was less need or desire to live in the city. Restaurants and bars were shut down. Theaters were closed. Public events with large groups of people were banned. The social world that people lived for in New York City was dead. Far and wide, the streets of NYC were empty. Perhaps it had never been this empty?

Omnicron

By May 2022, another perspective came alive. Omincron, a variant of COVID-19, was a more effective way to build the immune system than the booster shot. If you focus on building up the power of your immune system and practice appropriate hygiene, you can reduce your chances of getting it. So why not say, "I'm not waiting for a vaccine or living my life in fear of something that may not hurt me. Instead, I'm going to fortify my immune system and avoid large numbers of people in small spaces, and if I get it, I will manage it like any other sickness."

People who are most vulnerable to the virus

People with a weakened immune system, obese people, and people over 65 with existing health conditions are some of the most vulnerable to the virus. These people want to avoid the virus as much as possible by isolating and quarantining. If they have to go out, they should use masks and avoid getting within 6 feet of another person, especially indoors.

If I get the virus, can I get it again?

A question arose: "If I get the virus, can I get it again, or do I have permanent immunity?" If I get it the second time, will it be as bad as the first? I kept looking for the answers and couldn't find them. Eventually, John Sutcliffe explained that COVID-19 is similar to the flu virus; It mutates quickly. If you have one mutation of the virus, the vaccine is tailored to kill one variation of the virus and may not work for another variation of the virus. So, if you get the virus, you can get it again. A friend of mine who had the Coronavirus and nearly died from it said the worse you get it, the better your immune system is. He said the virus will not be so intense if he gets it again. Some people got the virus and had no symptoms. Do they have permanent immunity? If their immune system weakens, they could respond poorly to the virus. So you can keep getting the Coronavirus. If you have been vaccinated or had the virus, there is a good chance that you will not get extreme symptoms. Your immune system has been upgraded to the point where it can destroy the virus.

Just get the virus and get it over with.

The virus can not be avoided. Eventually, it will return in another form, and you will get it. The best one could do is to prevent it and build the immune system. If it comes around and I get it, I won't have any symptoms. It may not be worse than the flu, but as many people may not know, it kills 10-40,000 people annually. It's a number we are used to or don't talk about, or it's uncommon for someone we know to die from the flu unless they are older. Other than reducing anxiety, getting the virus to get over it is probably a bad idea. There needs to be more to gain. If you wait, you could get the vaccine, preventing getting drastically sick. Even if you are healthy, the virus can kill you.

Anti-vaccine arguments:

If you are against the vaccine, you won't be taking it and may not do anything to prevent its spread. Some say the vaccine is an experimental drug. The following are arguments against taking the vaccine:

The vaccine has not been adequately tested, so it is not safe.

Corporations and nations have made this vaccine to control people and make money.

The vaccine has too many side effects.

The vaccine will not work because the virus will mutate.

If the vaccine harms people, there's no way to hold corporations and nations accountable.

More than a few stories came out about people who were against the vaccine or denied the extent of the problem of the virus. Some of those people died from the virus. Other people said the vaccine made them sick and killed people.

Arguments for the vaccine:

The vaccine will provoke the immune system to produce antibodies against the virus.

The vaccine will blunt the virus's impact so that it does not damage or destroy the body's respiratory, immune, gastrointestinal, nervous, and other systems.

The vaccine will increase the number of people who will not get seriously sick from the virus, leading to herd immunity.

The vaccine will lead to fewer people going to the hospital, missing work, and not taking care of their families.

The vaccine will reduce the number of people who get seriously ill and die from the virus, which will improve the quality of life for many people.

Not getting the vaccine will lead to a collapse of the healthcare system, which would be overwhelmed with patients, leading to another level of catastrophe.

Developing and using vaccines will advance healthcare everywhere as the vaccine advances the experience and knowledge of combating pandemics.

Chapter 6

Housing

Housing

As the pandemic set in, the conditions for housing changed. People who lost jobs and income had to move with friends, family, or the street. The government wanted to prevent the spread of the virus with the eviction moratorium. It may have worked for some people. In some houses, people move in when a vacant room appears. Deadbeats, drug addicts, and criminals are always on the lookout for a cheap or spare room. Some know the housing laws enough to get months or years of free housing. Some help out and only do a slight damage. Others openly defy the rules and the law. They beat people, steal, do drugs, break doors and windows, and steal anything they can turn into money, including the boiler that heats their water and their house. The eviction moratorium provided some economic breathing room for people who work day and night and still can't pay the bills. Some received unemployment, which may have paid more than what they usually make. This was more fuel for the great resignation. For many, the eviction moratorium meant shelter from the pandemic and ruthless capitalism that required more money to live than they could make.

Eviction Moratorium

Governments enacted an eviction moratorium. The Centers for Disease Control (CDC) stopped evictions from September 2020 to August 2021. Local and state governments extended that for another 6-9 months. The government stopped doing evictions if you couldn't pay rent. Suddenly, landlords lost control of their properties. How could they pay taxes and insurance and maintain the property without income? When some tenants find out they don't have to pay, they will take advantage for as long as possible, even if it means having an eviction on their record. Some tenants kept paying rent, but others knew that the courts would not make them pay. For some, it meant free housing until the government came with a gun to evict them. Some took care of the property, and others used it for a shooting gallery, commercial theft, selling drugs, and prostitution. Landlords provided shelter for:

- People on a fixed income and older people.
- Anyone who claimed that they could not pay.
- People who couldn't afford to live.

Imagine losing your job, the rent is due, and people in your family are sick and dying from the virus. For many, the moratorium provided relief from the stress of the pandemic, but the relief was temporary. Even in the most liberal states, the moratorium didn't last much longer than January 2022. Landlords could claim they helped the country through the pandemic by providing free housing. Neither the government nor tenants gave a public thank you to the landlords.

ERAP

The Emergency Rental Assistance Program (ERAP) provided money to landlords to pay rent for those who couldn't pay during the pandemic. Landlords and tenants had to fill out paperwork to qualify. The program paid rent for those who lost their job during the pandemic. New York State was very slow to pay landlords. Texas was the opposite. Some landlords wouldn't cooperate, and some tenants did nothing. For the deadbeats, criminals, and drug addicts, it was a green light for free housing. The government obligated the tenants to pay during the pandemic, but there was little enforcement. Unless the barrel of a gun was at the door, many would not leave. At most, they would appear in court. Just showing up a few times was enough to get you 2-4 months or years of free housing. You didn't need to bring a lawyer; just show up. In New York, getting rent money from some tenants during the pandemic was impossible. Some had money, but why pay when no one was there to enforce the rules? For the landlords that did get paid, ERAP money provided the means for them to continue being an economic engine in the local economy. Landlords pay large amounts for taxes, insurance, plumbers, electricians, carpenters, lawyers, and accountants. Without ERAP money, some landlords had a very tough time, and some gave up and quit. For many landlords, ERAP provided barely enough money to keep them from going out of business.

Time and money for renovation

Building supply stores did well during the pandemic. Without jobs and with government assistance, some were able to do home improvement projects that had not been possible for a long time. People renovated kitchens, bathrooms, and bedrooms and upgraded their houses. Some seized the opportunity to improve their housing and watch the appreciation soar.

Housing and commuting

Work from home expanded during the pandemic. Commuters who spent 1-5 hours commuting daily worked from home. With students at home, some in smaller homes and apartments, competition for internet bandwidth increased. People needed a spot in the house without people having multiple conversations simultaneously. A teacher could lecture students in one room, and a parent could work online in the next room. The house became the workplace and school overnight. Suddenly, the possibilities of the internet expanded as people realized they could share their work, life, hobbies, support groups, and medicine without leaving their homes. Their house now saved them time and money, but with a price. With more activity in the house, stress rose. Home became more active and focused, but also more stressful and deadly.

Houses with the virus

If someone in the house got the virus, everyone was likely exposed, and everyone would get it. That's the logic, yet in more than a few households, some people got it and some people didn't, and in some homes, more than one died from the virus. If you thought the virus was a hoax or a government plot, there was no reason to take it seriously. Wearing a mask, washing hands, or social distancing wasn't crucial for your health. According to the Centers for Disease Control (CDC), more than 10,000 people died at home from the virus. For people with the most risk, those over 65, or those with severe heart and lung problems or compromised immune systems, the virus could strike hard and fast and kill quickly. Many didn't make it, even in hospitals with the best equipment and drugs. With the hospitals at capacity, many were sent home to die.

People have accepted the virus, and some take precautions, but the US is not an authoritarian country.

I'm writing this paragraph in June 2022. People have accepted that the virus will be around and that we should go on living. Masks are required in transit and transit stations. However, it's common to see people without masks. The trains are more strict than the buses. Some bus drivers don't wear masks. Ultimately, I got into more trouble for bringing a bicycle on a bus than not wearing a mask. I wore a mask and put one on for the conductors to see, but one conductor refused to let me on the train with a bicycle. We don't stop people from eating meat, smoking, or drinking alcohol. Society accepts these activities without requiring that they live a healthy life so they can avoid the leading causes of death: heart disease and cancer. More people have a sense of what the risks are and how dangerous the virus is. Many people have been vaccinated or had the virus and have some immunity from another virus variation. People don't live forever. If you don't live now, what good is life?

Mask mandates aren't enforced as the pandemic subsides.

The authorities are not enforcing the mask mandate like they used to. This is due, in part, because of the change in the laws. Mask mandates were struck down in some of the courts. Many people say the masks don't prevent the virus. Most may not wear or use the mask properly. Some say only an N95-type mask may stop the virus, but they don't know how it spreads. If the virus spreads like smoke and leaves particles on everything, people may get it by touching something with their hands and transferring it to their mouth or nose. This may be a minimal amount, which may or may not make a difference. The immune system may kill a small amount of the virus if a person is healthy.

So, get the virus and be done with it?

I never expected an educated person to be against vaccines or mask mandates. They may have a healthy distrust of the government or corporations. Another perspective is that "I'm healthy and not likely to get the virus, and if I do, so what? I'll get over it, build my immunity, and become stronger. I don't have to go around day and night worried about and afraid of getting the virus." The vaccine is an experimental drug that was not adequately tested. Government workers responsible for ensuring the vaccine is ready for public use have resigned.

Corporations and governments with much to gain from the vaccine may push people to accept that it works.

When the pandemic first hit, New York state quickly shut down economic activity that could spread the virus. Bars, restaurants, and large gatherings were shut down, especially indoors. The city became a ghost town overnight. The government-controlled business and human activity in the biggest way: stopping all activity, but that didn't stop the virus. That was only possible if you did what the Chinese did.

Chapter 7

Racism

The pandemic provoked intense responses. People in the United States were looking for someone to blame. Media reports and some government officials pointed fingers at China, which was an obvious scapegoat. The virus may or may not have originated in China. Some reports indicate that it was in Italy or Europe at nearly the same time as China. Some people in the US who were looking for a scapegoat for the failed policies of the United States were quick to blame China. This led to an explosion of hatred and violence against people who looked Asian or like they could be from China. As Trump denied a problem with the virus, he told the country that the virus came from China. This gave the green light to his henchman, who went on a rampage around the country.

Documented racist attacks on Asians during the pandemic

Racially motivated violence against Asians and Pacific Islanders rose significantly during the pandemic. A variety of polls indicate the following:

The FBI has documented a 77% increase in hate crimes against Asian Americans from 2019 to 2020.

More than 9000 anti-Asian hate incidents were self-reported between March 2020 and June 2021 to Stop AAIP Hate,

The people experiencing this hate and discrimination are from a diverse range of people in the US, including Hawaii and Pacific islanders. Some of them don't speak English, so they cannot communicate any incidents that may have happened to them. One poll indicated that over half of those surveyed said they often or sometimes do not feel safe in public. One in 7 people from that poll said that they felt discrimination or threats from people who thought that if you are Asian, you will have the virus. Polls indicate that the reason for the racism is that Asians are used as scapegoats for the failure of Donald Trump and the Republicans to keep Americans safe during the pandemic. The president and his politicians, the Republicans, failed to provide means to keep Americans safe during the pandemic. To draw attention away from their failure, they said that people should blame the Chinese and Asians for the problem. Research has indicated that it is unclear where the virus came from.

Documenting, Tracing, and responding to attacks

Victims, activists, and many Asians want the government to take action:

Provide ways to report anti-Asian hate speech, discrimination, and attacks.

Track groups and individuals responsible for anti-Asian attacks and bias.

Respond to reports, prosecute, and arrest people responsible for Asian American attacks.

Polls indicate that Asian Americans do not feel like they can trust the police to treat them with courtesy and respect. Asian Americans support increasing funding for police training to identify and respond to anti-Asian American Asian and Pacific Islander bias.

Discrimination and racist attacks have consequences, including:

Reduced sense of safety and security.

Reduce participation in public events and social activities.

Increased anxiety, fear, depression, and mental health services.

More people are dropping out of the system.

The following are potential solutions to reduce racism in the United States.

Identify and report hate crimes to the FBI.

Report and respond to bullying and harassment in schools and universities.

Educate the public to report, identify, and report bias and hate crimes against Asian Americans and Pacific Islanders.

Stop assuming Asian Americans are not Americans as much as any other American.

Identify racist and discriminating language, which leads to stigmatizing, scapegoating, and impeding a unifying response.

Increase ways to report anti-Asian attacks, track discrimination, and hold accountable those responsible for the problem.

Minneapolis police officer murders George Floyd.

During the summer of 2020, demonstrations and riots jolted the country. On May 25, 2020, Derek Chauvin, a white police officer in Minneapolis, apprehended and murdered George Floyd. Floyd, a black man, was detained for a minor infraction of the law. A girl videotaped the event. Viewers across the world saw a man go from life to death as a group of police officers and people on the street watched and did nothing to stop the attack. With a glaring and brutal bluntness, an unarmed, innocent man was killed. How could one officer do this without other officers stopping it, and what should have the people who were watching the murder? Imagine how much trouble you would get into if you tried to stop that cop from committing murder.

Murder triggers a national response.

The murder erupted in a national response. Demonstrations in Los Angeles, New York, Portland, and Minneapolis continued throughout the summer. Buildings were looted and burnt. Many were killed and injured. One push was to stop funding for the police and shut the police force down. Efforts in Minneapolis started with a bang but went bust, as many feared what would happen if the police were dismantled. Would white people have to give up their power and privilege? National Public Radio reported that armed groups were forming as vigilantes believed that the police were not doing their job. The fires and break-ins terrified the shop owners, patrons, and local people who didn't want to see their neighborhood burned down.

White Supremacy

Trump blamed immigrants for the problems of the white working class. He exploited white working-class disenchantment after decades of wage losses from union breaking, automation, outsourcing, and immigrants. After Obama demonstrated that a non-white person could be president, many whites, including women, saw the writing on the wall. They were afraid of losing their privileges. White suburban women voted for Trump over Hillary Clinton, which shocked many people. Wouldn't a white woman want another white woman to be president? Especially a woman who had been so close to the presidency. Trump praised white people over others, denigrated non-white people, and helped racist authoritarians in positions of power to carry out attacks on non-white people. Blaming the Chinese for the pandemic led to a long wave of anti-Asian attacks. Blacks were pitted against Asians as Asians were characterized as the model minority and blacks as the opposite. The open and callous bigotry broadcast by the white house was echoed and spread around the world by the dominant media.

Americans against bigotry respond.

Many were disgusted by the bigotry chaining the country to a backward status while undermining US efforts to improve human rights around the world. The country desperately needed a leader to unite people and subdue the pandemic. Instead, Trump spread fuel on the fires of hatred, misogyny, and racism. Many called for the police to be abolished or reformed. Measures can be taken to control the spread of hatred, discrimination, and attacks against people of difference, including:

Calling out and denouncing leaders who send bigoted messages.

Denounce bigotry, including racist, sexist, and homophobic statements and actions.

Poll groups that are victims of bigoted attacks.

Overhaul the system that supports white supremacy.

Minneapolis

The police killing of a black man, which showed a man alive and dead the next second, sent a title wave of shock, anger, and grief around the world. As the world watched, time stood still as the pain swept the nation. How could all those people watch it happen and do nothing? What kind of system could produce such madness? For many, it was nothing new. A routine traffic stop could result in someone getting beaten or killed for no reason. The system maintained inequality and made an example to terrify the rest into compliance. With the image in your mind, would you feel safe around the police?

The US enforces bigotry throughout society. The patriarchy is codified into the laws that started the country. At the time, it was accepted, just like the prisons, the war machine, and slavery. An epidemic of racial violence, especially against Americans of African and Asian descent, continues to strike families, friends, and communities everywhere. Senseless killing destroys confidence in the police and the system. Why pay taxes if the police come and terrorize the neighborhood? Why call the police if they use it as an excuse to beat and harass people? Human rights groups have called out bigots and bullies in the police force. With the rise of Donald Trump and the extreme right, the role of the police came under scrutiny. For years, there have been reports of extreme right-leaning people infiltrating the police force and using the police force to coerce and bully people. The police uniform became a cover for bullying and bigotry at an institutional level.

Chapter 8

More Time

As people settled into the pandemic, some began to realize an opportunity. With more time and fewer places to go, people took action. Renovation projects, planting trees and bushes, and that book I always wanted to write, well, now I have time for it. The luxury of time was a significant benefit during the pandemic. Most had never had a couple of months or more of a break from work, and yes, all the government payments made life a lot easier for many people. It was like entering another world that only those with money or those willing to live with few expenses could afford. This lifestyle is possible in a cooperative living situation, but most have yet to learn what it is or how to get it. The idea of living with less money to have more time was an unknown equation. The dominant idea of success is a house with a backyard, two cars, a garage, and some money for savings. Time is not part of the equation.

I was living outside the system to generate more freedom.

It's possible to work less and have more time. Many things people are brainwashed into needing are not necessary. Living without a car in the US can be challenging, but it can work well in progressive urban areas prioritizing transit, bicycle, and pedestrian infrastructure. Cities with good public transit and bike lanes make cars obsolete. This can cut the cost of living while improving the standard of living. Some people find, grow, or learn to eat wild food. This can cut expenses. Some people shop on the curb as they go home. What you find is free and another way to avoid the rat race and help to stop global warming. All of these activities can increase your time. These activities don't give you the pleasure of shopping and buying on Amazon. However, they can give you more freedom to live the life you want. During the pandemic, some people had more time to live without spending money. As people develop habits outside of production and consumption, they can liberate themselves from the dictates of capitalism and the state.

Commuting during the pandemic

People who went out to bars, restaurants, and theaters had less reason to be in the city. Many had houses outside New York City on Long Island or north of the town. As remote work became the go-to solution for many, labor was no longer tied to offices in the city. Living anywhere with an internet connection and a job was now possible. Commuting was not needed anymore. That could add 30 minutes to 4 hours to people's free time. Without the hassle of commuting, the standard of living increased for many as they no longer had to spend their time, energy, and money on commuting.

I'd trade money for time any day of the week. I'd use my skills to make what money can't buy. With more than enough and too many things available for free, who wants to work so much to purchase consumer goods, use something for a little while, and then discard it? This creates an infinite wasteland that puts the planet on a collision course with extinction. The economic slowdown was a welcome relief from the endless push of the capitalist economy.

Time or money

Perhaps the rat race pace of pre-pandemic life was impossible to be aware of. Many had yet to learn of anything else besides the nonstop work-to-live grind. The dominant system pushes nonstop production and consumption, but is this a life worth living? For some, debt became the ball and chain of indentured servitude. The more debt you have, the more you have to work. Endless debt that can't be paid off requires endless work without getting ahead or a way to escape.

The reset button for the malaise of production.

When you get sick, your body shuts down to make time to heal, to shut down the system, and to get enough rest. People push their limits; something breaks, and it's time to shut it down. The global production and consumption machine is so large with so much mass that just getting it to slow down significantly could take a long time. The wrecking ball of climate change may generate a slowdown in the capitalist extinction machine. The pandemic was like a global reset button, but before global warming could slow down, it sped up and continued to increase.

Children stopped going to school and attended classes using the Internet.

Without the means to keep children safe at school, most schools were shut down during the pandemic. The government's solution to keep children safe while providing classes was to do online learning. With the Internet and computers in most households, the school systems were set up for students to take courses online. An internet connection and computers were required. Most families had this setup, and those without could use the computers at school. Families with large numbers of children had some challenges to work through. Perhaps it wouldn't have been a big problem if each student had room and enough resources. Conflicts were inevitable, with parents working from home and children going to school at home. What if the Internet didn't work? Or what if they didn't have enough computers? Even with enough hardware and bandwidth, schedules may collide. Somehow, people made it work. Parents worried less about their children getting to school on time. Some children didn't leave their beds. Like the adults, children didn't have to commute to school. This saved time, energy, and money, but the family could have a big crisis if the virus got into the house. With all the people at home in a small area, it's likely that if one person got the virus, all of them got it. Not commuting to school saved children time but added more responsibility for the parents. Missing school was very damaging to the mental health of the child. This broke some children, who had anxiety and depression and turned to drugs and sometimes worse. Overall, not going to school meant more time at home for the child, but that was not worth the price they had to pay. Many children were quite miserable at home, and not establishing and maintaining friendships was a massive blow to their state of mind. They felt insecure, like there was a huge part of childhood and growing up that was as necessary as good food that the pandemic had taken away, and now it was eating a dark hole in their reason to live.

Chapter 9

Government Response

Donald Trump was president during the pandemic. One promise he made before the pandemic was that he would rid the country of the regulations that stopped businesses from making money. In 2017, Trump proposed to cut the budget for the pandemic response team and the Centers for Disease Control. A bipartisan group of legislators, including some Republicans, refused to cut the budget. Eventually, Trump dismantled a government that could help the country respond to a pandemic. All previous presidents after George W. Bush, including Republican presidents, supported a federal pandemic response. Trump was running the country like a business. He had no experience in government. Most jobs require previous experience in a similar job. Trump exploited a loophole. For Trump, people are expendable as a piece of toilet paper. He has a long history of screwing people who work for him. The system put him in place to advance Trump, capitalism, and white power.

Without a pandemic response team, the government couldn't prevent the spread of the virus.

With the pandemic response team crushed by President Trump, the government lost a way to fight the pandemic. As soon as the reports came out, the US government could have started to prepare people to avoid and control the virus. Instead, the government did nothing and let the virus spread through NYC and beyond. Prevention is a foreign word if there is no public health care system. In the for-profit system, people will make more money if the virus spreads. They lose money if they prevent the virus from spreading. Few say that healthcare employees work solely to make money without regard for the health and safety of their patients. However, the system as a whole differs from the individuals who operate the system. The rules are set with government regulation. Regulations don't prioritize preventive medical systems. Governments that pay for public healthcare know that the way to minimize expenses is to maximize preventative healthcare. Typically, this is not a concern for Republicans; instead, they are most interested in setting up the conditions for the hospitals to bank as much money as possible.

The government provided money for qualified people to live during the pandemic.

Money for unemployed people

The government provided pandemic relief benefits for those who qualified, which didn't include undocumented workers. The government made the following payments.

1. March 2020: $1200 for adults and $600 for children. A family of four with an income under $112,000 could get $3400.

2. In late 2020, the government gave out $600 for each adult and $600 for each child. The income caps were reduced below $75,000 for single people.

3. In early 2021, the government paid $1400 to each adult and $1400 to each dependent.

The government has paid the following:

$411 billion in payments to individuals

$362 billion in payments to state, local, and tribal governments

$203 billion unemployment extension payments

$173 billion tax incentives

$174 billion for health measures

$170 billion for education

$301 billion for other programs

The Centers for Disease Control

The CDC's goal has been to stop the spread of the virus. It collects information about the virus and vaccines to track side effects and find ways to limit the spread of the virus. It also works with healthcare providers and frontline workers to develop vaccine programs.

The CDC:

Publishes documents to help hospitals ensure they have the equipment, supplies, and information required to control the virus.

It makes programs to predict the number of ventilators and intensive care units needed to help patients.

Advises businesses, communities, and schools on how to prepare for and move through the pandemic.

Help schools make decisions on whether or not they should do in-person learning.

Guide businesses that want to let people work from home.

It helps schools respond to a COVID outbreak and makes planning guides for organizations, households, and people hosting large gatherings.

Increase unemployment benefits, Medicaid, and food programs.

Businesses must provide sick and medical leave and free coronavirus testing.

$500 billion was paid to large corporations and governments to assist businesses that work on national security issues and distressed areas of the economy. Loans to small businesses to avoid large-scale layoffs of workers, 290 billion direct payments to families, 150 billion to health care providers, 82 billion for schools

The government downplayed the problems with the virus to make the government look better.

Some say that by downplaying the virus's problem, it spread because people didn't take it seriously or take enough preventative measures. The government restricted reporting, so the Centers for Disease Prevention and Control couldn't be honest with the public. People thought the virus was less of a problem than it was. Censoring experts made it impossible for the government to give accurate and life-saving information to the public.

Uncle Sam protects profits over people.

Delays by the government gave the virus more time to spread. Staying ahead of the virus and prevention are nearly foreign concepts in the US, where hospitals exist for profit first and patients second. So, the government let the virus spread, which quickly killed 20,000 people in New York City. That was the tip of the iceberg, as 1 million more had to give their lives to ensure the system continues profiting. The CDC developed its test for the virus, even though they could have used the one approved by the World Health Organization (WHO). The CDC test was flawed and had to be corrected, which gave the virus more time to infect more people. Some say the CDC was too slow to approve the new tests. The time-tested methods of stopping a virus, testing, tracing contacts, and quarantining were not followed. However, countries like Vietnam, South Korea, and New Zealand have reduced the impact of the virus by using these methods. Information about using a mask was contradictory, making it less effective. Trump refused to wear a mask and belittled people who wore a mask and followed prudent protocol. Even though the government poured money into people's pockets, it failed to protect them from the virus, which resulted in 1 million deaths and countless others who needlessly had to suffer through the virus.

Better at home or in the hospital?

The hospitals had to treat a warload of patients. They had to do this without the proper equipment, procedures, and drugs. Imagine being a nurse, doctor, or frontline worker who had to work without a mask or adequate equipment. Medical and frontline workers could quickly get the virus and spread it around. The virus could have concentrated in various medical facilities, especially if they lacked proper ventilation, sanitation procedures, supplies, and equipment. It may have been similar to a war zone situation. The patients could go to the hospital, and there was a good chance they would not come out alive. The virus could get them and some other illnesses in the hospital, or with doctors sick, tired, and overworked, they may make more mistakes.

People who live alone have less chance of passing the virus to someone else. Some people are used to staying home. They would still need help getting food and treatment, but I knew someone with complications: obesity, heart and lung issues, and over 60. They told him to go home, where he nearly died more than once and survived. He was a squatter used to challenging conditions. He had almost no help at home. It's hard to say if he would've survived in the hospital. When you are sick, taking care of yourself is very difficult. Some people who are short on money must work when they are ill. You must get your food, see doctors on your own, and pick up the medicine. When you go to the doctor, you are giving your life to the doctor. The doctor will do procedures and prescribe drugs to help you heal. This seems like a huge advantage. So, you would be much better off in the hospital, but that may not be the case in a pandemic.

Government response to the Coronavirus.

Governments in the US responded in different ways. Trump denied that the virus was a problem and dismantled the federal government pandemic response team in 2018. The government should have taken immediate action to provide personal protective equipment, medical supplies, and ventilators to hospitals. Taking immediate action to educate the public more thoroughly could have saved many lives. People didn't know much about the virus. Leaders of healthcare in the government could have educated the press and public so that people could reduce the spread and impact of the virus. Local governments had to provide health care for people with the virus. The healthcare system was quickly overwhelmed with more patients than supplies, ventilators, nurses, and doctors. Many people needing medical treatment were turned away and had to fend for themselves. Some died at home, and some survived. Not being in the hospital could have been an advantage for people. Trump's government killed a million people as it failed to inform and protect the public from the virus. Consider what happened in China, a country with four times the population of the US, had 6,000 deaths from the Coronavirus, while over 1 million died in the US.

Chapter 10

Transport

In March 2020, the New York State governor, Andrew Cuomo, shut down non-essential businesses. Some commuter buses continued until April 2020. After that, it became nearly impossible to get from New York City to Newburgh, NY, a distance of 60 miles. The last month before the buses stopped running, many buses had less than five people in them. In May 2022, commuter buses have yet to come close to what they were before the pandemic.

Too much new infrastructure

Large park and ride lots with transit connections are located near Woodbury Commons, 60 miles north of New York City. These are big money projects with lots of pavement. The construction has been going on for years before the pandemic. During the beginning and ending months of the pandemic, from March 2020 to mid-January 2022, many buses and trains were nearly empty. It was spooky and luxurious. I kept riding as long as the buses ran. Most people were frightened or had no reason to travel. The traffic picked up very slowly, but it's not close to what it used to be. If commuters stop using the buses and people refuse to commute to work, the government may have built a lot of roads and parking lots that won't be used often. This is a big waste.

Bicycling in New York City

Before the pandemic, bicycling in NYC, particularly between Houston Street and 42nd Street, was easiest around 4 am, but by 5:30 am, the pace would increase very quickly. In most of these areas, traffic can get quite intense. At the beginning of the moratorium, there was little bicycle traffic. That changed very quickly as people ordered more takeout food. This increased the number of electric bikes used for delivery. Bicycling in New York City is probably the most dangerous way to get around. Many different types of one or two-wheel electric vehicles operate in the area. Many go in any direction they want. Parked car drivers may open their doors and hit a bicycle while riding by. This has happened to me four times over 20 years. Usually, I walk away, but not without injuries. Bicycle riding in New York City may have increased to levels larger than before the pandemic. The bike lanes can be hazardous. If you make the slightest mistake, you could be in an accident. The accident could be minor or major. Only a few very cautious people can ride in New York City without an accident.

There's less traffic.

Even on a Friday afternoon on a sunny day, it's a quick ride through the Lincoln Tunnel that connects New Jersey to New York City. Before the pandemic, drivers often waited at least 20 minutes. The traffic would be backed up and moving a couple of yards per minute. It was pretty frustrating and an example of what commuters have to put up with. As four or five lanes of vehicles are idling, the pollution concentrates. The pandemic reduced traffic from New Jersey to New York City, but the Lincoln Tunnel is still quite busy, and it may not be long until vehicles clog up the freeway, just like it used to be.

Bus Transport takes a big hit.

While some commuter trains kept running, the bus traffic faded. At the beginning of the pandemic, most of the buses stopped. Many buses had less than five riders. The second most popular vacation spot in New York, Woodbury Commons, shut down. As more people worked from home, less people used the buses. Two years after the pandemic, commuter bus companies are struggling. Buses run on a limited schedule. As they attempted to operate more routes, the risk for the company increased. A bus that holds 45 people but has only 5-7 people on it is a waste of resources. Hopefully, artificial intelligence will figure out how transit can operate more efficiently. A bus company can't operate with that level of riders. Recently, Shortline Bus Company filed for bankruptcy. People still depend on these buses. When there's no bus, riders are in a challenging position. Many can't work, attend school, or function without adequate transit.

Sidewalk Sheds

During the pandemic, restaurants were shut down in New York City (NYC). Gradually, the city looked for ways to keep them open and keep people safe from the pandemic. An opportunity opened since the traffic was low and streets were used less. Why not use the parking spaces in front of a restaurant for outdoor seating? The city allowed restaurants to build sheds in the parking spaces in front of the restaurant. Many variations of the sheds appeared. Some used clear panels on the sides and tops. Others used wood. Some were adorned with plants. Others were flimsy and open and blew down in the wind. All manor of color and style were explored. Perhaps these were most common in Manhattan, especially in the East Village. Possibly twice a month, you'd hear a report of a car smashing into the sheds and injuring someone. People would be breathing vehicle exhaust and hearing the sound of traffic as they were supposed to enjoy the food. The sheds had to be built loose enough to allow enough ventilation to minimize the spread of the virus. The sheds were a significant expense for restaurants. Now, they had to make a small building on the side and maintain it. Some had heaters inside. This may require a significant upgrade of the power system. By 2024, many sidewalk sheds had been removed.

Struggle for bicycles on a commuter train.

The Hudson Line, an MTA commuter train, follows the eastern edge of the Hudson River. It's rare for a railway to have such a privileged place alongside a beautiful river. So I locked my bicycle on the train and was going to take a seat, and he came through the door. A large guy with a train operator's uniform entered the train and told me I had to leave. He told me bicycles were not allowed on the train. I began to argue. The train was 20% full. They called it a peak-hour train, but the train was nearly empty. With few riders, what sense does it make to deny service because someone uses a bicycle? There were no safety issues. I know because I asked. I had been using the train for many months without a problem. All the other conductors allowed bicycles on the train. There was no other way for me to get to Newburgh. I was working to make affordable housing. The whole gesture was an authoritarian routine. The police backed him up and told me I had to leave.

No transit, no work

Finally, I gave in and left. Yes, I needed to get to Beacon as soon as possible. I had to meet with Frank, who would help me with the carpentry. Now, that could not happen. How would I get to Beacon? No commuter buses were going from New York to Newburgh. That would mean that I have one less hour to work. That meant I would have 2.5 hours to work and then return. My commute is 2.5 hours one way. I was freaked out and didn't know what to do, so I went to the service counter and asked if I could complain. They handed me the form, and I filled it out and returned it. I was still too excited and anxious; how would I get to work? Will another authoritarian stop me from using the train because I have a bicycle or because they read the rules and now say I can't go on the train?

Anxiety into action

I walked around the Grand Central Terminal and was flipping out. Finally, I asked the ticket window person to give me a copy of the Metropolitan Transit Authority (MTA) bicycle policy rules. To my surprise, happiness, and vindication, I read that my bicycle was allowed. Armed with this document, I would confront the man. The next day, I rode my bike from the east village to Grand Central. Not knowing what was going to happen, I kept going anyway. The trains are nearly empty and have lost many riders after the pandemic; why are they turning down customers? The worst they could do is deny me service, right?

Confronting the police and conductor

I had no idea what was going to happen. The day before, the conductor refused to let me use the train. He said the rules didn't allow it. I had been riding during peak hours before, and all the conductors had no problem with my bicycle. Armed with the document proving that I could ride the train, I confronted him and told him the rules were clear: I could ride on the train. After I disagreed with him, he immediately called the police. Six police officers were there in a minute and came toward me. Five went to talk to the conductor. One came to talk to me. The police officer explained that the conductor has authority and that sometimes they are audited by people who pose as passengers to check the conductor's performance. I explained the document and told him he had to allow me on the train. He refused. Again, the police backed up the conductor, even when the conductor was wrong. So, I gave up on getting on that train but wouldn't give up my fight.

Day 3 arrived. I was going to see if I could get on the train, even though the conductor and the police, the authoritarians, said that I couldn't take my bicycle on an empty train. I would sneak into the train the back way and see if I could get in without him making a fuss. As I approached the back of the train, I saw the authoritarian conductor. I had no idea what was going to happen. Surprisingly, he told me I could ride the train if I put my bicycle in the back car with no one in it. He explained that until the MTA clarified its rules, I was allowed to use the train. It was a victory. A few moments later, I saw other bicyclers getting on the train and putting them in the empty car in the back. Now, we will see what happens. Will the MTA cling to its outdated rules? Or will it do the right thing and allow people with bicycles to use the trains?

Lucky for me, I never saw that conductor again. None of the other conductors ever hassled me, not one of them. He confessed that he was in the military and liked to follow rules.

Transportation, especially commuter transport, was severely affected by the pandemic. Many people stopped going to work and started working from home. Other people depended on that transit, but now it was not operating. Some transit lines shut down entirely after the pandemic and may never be available again. People who depend on that transport will have to find alternatives; for many, it will mean they have to invest in a vehicle, stop working, or stop visiting people and places.

Chapter 11

Mental Health

The pandemic of 2019 challenged people in many ways. People lost friends, family members, and jobs. Many suffered from a wide variety of mental health issues, including anxiety, depression, and suicide. The virus wreaked havoc on the whole body. In general, the ability of people to function went down as the pandemic swept the country.

Everything and nothing

Imagine the impact when someone close is not around anymore. Something inside is not there anymore. The silence goes on forever. Life becomes something else. In 2021, government sources reported that over 400,000 people died from COVID-19. This strange little thing enters the body, and time changes. It keeps going and stops at the same time. Big waves of nothing and emptiness envelop the space. Nothing and everything is the same and different at the same time. In the numbness of it all, people keep going; step by step, people keep moving.

Facing the crash

Some faced the crash head-on and got through it. The flu times ten was no joke for those lucky enough to make it through. Unless you were near death, the hospitals would not let you in. The virus exploits weakness. Alone, your chances of making it through sunk. With help, people could help you with medicine, herbs, comfort, and distraction. Not knowing if you would make it or be another number generates anxiety, stress, and emotional pain.

Losing a loved one produces mental health problems.

Death from any cause can generate anxiety, depression, fear, frustration, numbness, and sadness. When someone dies, people must decide what to do with the body. Some use a funeral home and casket, which cost $4,000-10,000 for the most basic service. A cremation can cost between $700-10,000. If you donate to a university or medical center, they may cover the cost. If the will is contested, the consequences of death can go on for years without resolution. What will be done with the house, bank accounts, and endless amounts of paper, books, clothes, and other items? Many people have loaded their lives with too much already.

Losing a job may produce anxiety.

Losing a job generates anxiety about whether or not you will have enough money to live a decent life. Will I still have a place to live, food, and access to a life worth living? The pandemic was a new cause of death. We were used to the other causes. What will happen to the economy? Will it create more jobs after the pandemic recedes? Finding coherent information during the pandemic was quite a challenge.

Uncertainty about the virus generated mental anguish.

Like most people and businesses, the public needed to be better informed about the virus. How can I avoid it? How can I prevent it? If I get the vaccine, do I have immunity for the rest of my life? Some epidemiologists and well-informed people knew the basic answers to these questions, but most didn't know. The media focused on a single issue, like whether or not people have to wear masks.

The stigma of mental illness prevents people from talking about it.

If your family and friends only brag about what they have done, they may not be so open about their weaknesses. Mental illness stops people from taking action. Negative thoughts and language reduce motivation to get out of bed and take action. "Why should I do this? Nothing will happen from it anyway." People don't want to look vulnerable around people they are competitive with. Admitting that I'm depressed will drive people away from me. People who are depressed can make people around them depressed. Keeping motivated and positive requires effort.

The quackery about the virus

Ideas spread far and wide about the virus. Since it seems to have originated in China, some people thought it was a plot by the Chinese to take over the world. Others felt corporations and the government used it to control people and make money.

Many people may not know they have a mental illness.

If people aren't educated about mental illness, they may not know what it is or how to identify it. Mental illness doesn't have a physical form, such as a cut, bruise, or another physical injury. Denying it becomes easier if you are not familiar with it or know how to recognize it. Reading and talking about it may help. People who write down their symptoms and discuss them with people who have been through it may be better at identifying the virus. When people in power talk to the media about their mental health issues, it helps other people admit that they haven't been feeling well and that they may have the same problem. Sometimes, people don't realize what happened to them until decades later. People may not do so well without education, discussion, and therapy. K-12 could have ongoing education that includes mental health problems that they work through.

Many people don't have access to mental health care

Some estimates report that less than 8% of the US population has access to mental health care. Others say it's much higher. Medicaid pays for mental health treatment; many health care plans do the same. With suicide rates escalating and millions with mental health problems, the need for more care should not be underestimated.

In some families, going to a psychiatrist is new.

Some people don't trust psychiatry. They may not know that a psychiatrist has to become a doctor first, then advance with another degree focusing on psychiatry. That's a lot of institutional training. This is one reason why they are so expensive. Many low-income people would rather spend their money on housing and food. Some people don't like therapists because therapists may have a disdain for herbal approaches and dismiss using pot, LSD, or mushrooms. Others may dismiss a psychiatrist as someone who is there to integrate you into capitalism and become a good consumer. Non-privileged people may be used to doing things on their own and may not see a need for a therapist.

Poor nutrition

Many have yet to learn that eating and drinking affect your thoughts and feelings. A common misunderstanding is that fried food tastes good, so there's no need to worry or consider how it affects your state of mind. Not drinking water can lead to feelings that are similar to depression. Non-organic foods may contain fertilizers, pesticides, and herbicides. Reports indicate that highly processed foods may cause depression. These can damage your brain and how you interpret the world. If most of your thoughts are negative, you may be on a collision course with depression.

Lack of exercise may increase mental health problems

Exercise increases endorphins, which make you happy. With more strength, people gain the confidence to move heavy things, climb stairs, and get through accidents. As you improve your physical health, you gain confidence to engage in other things. When people get used to sitting on the couch too much, their options for physical activity may shrink.

The pandemic tested people's ability to adapt and survive like no other challenge. Except for a tiny amount of people, the pandemic was a complete surprise. With people getting sick and dying from a disease that had no cure, people could slide into a mental health crisis easily. Further shocks to everyday life occurred when the government shut down businesses, schools, and government services. Suddenly, the world was turned upside down. It was the biggest test many would endure, and some would not pass. School children suffered anxiety, depression, and substance abuse at alarming levels. Many others struggle to keep their life with family and friends. The pandemic brought a wave of mental health issues that many endured and survived.

Chapter 12

Work

Quickly after the big shutdown in March 2020, many people lost their jobs. Live entertainment venues, restaurants, bars, and theaters could not operate. Schools were closed, and workplaces shut down. Indoor gatherings with people close together had to stop meeting. The virus spread quickly in meat production plants. Workers were transmitting the virus. People on airplanes brought viruses from one country to another. Those on the front lines, nurses, doctors, and emergency workers, faced war zone-like stress and challenges. They could pass it on to other nurses, doctors, and patients if they got infected. Some slept in their cars for fear of bringing the virus home and killing their families. After many years of no vacation, the virus upended the work ethic of many who finally got a taste of living without the endless struggle of living from paycheck to paycheck after the government provided extended unemployment benefits.

Medical workers

Hospital workers faced the brutal impact of the pandemic. Only the sickest people were admitted to the hospital. Many suffered in their homes, and some didn't make it. Elective surgeries were put on hold, and hospitals had to separate Co-Vid patients from the rest of the patients. With nurses and doctors taking care of patients with the virus, they were likely to get the virus. Hospitals had to manage colossal emergencies with inadequate preparation, training, supplies, and equipment. Many on the front lines were given the cold shoulder by Trump, the president when they asked for more equipment to keep them safe while working. The stress and psychological toll of the virus pushed many towards complete breakdown. They were used to seeing their patients get better, not worse, and die. While the majority were safe at home, medical workers fought a war against the pandemic.

More people work from home.

A significant change, accelerated by the pandemic, was the expansion of the number of people working from home. Some people roamed the planet and still kept their jobs. All they needed was an internet connection. Others were tied down and worked from home. Many restaurant and bar workers lost their jobs. Being closer to family generated significant advantages. Parents could be around their children during the day and enjoy life without commuting. Working from home increased the time, energy, and money to commute. With some people committing 4 hours a day, the improvement in daily life was significant but offset by the challenges of the pandemic. If you were lucky not to get sick and die from the Coronavirus, perhaps you had a friend or relative who got it. For most, working from home provided more advantages than commuting to work every day.

Restaurants and Bars

Non-essential businesses, including restaurants, bars, and theaters, had to shut down. The government was in emergency mode. It may be erring on the side of safety over economic damage. Workers in the entertainment industry lost their jobs immediately. While the government provided unemployment benefits, undocumented workers didn't qualify. People living from paycheck to paycheck didn't lose their housing because of the eviction moratorium and received money from the government. This gave them some breathing room, but how can a business survive when the government takes control, shuts them down, and requires extensive and costly regulations?

Take-out food businesses expand.

People stayed at home. You could still buy groceries at the store, but some didn't want to take a chance. Some businesses seized the opportunity and expanded delivery service. The take-out food business boomed. With less traffic and less need for parking, the city legalized sidewalk sheds for restaurants. People could eat outside with less of a chance to spread the virus. Electric bike deliveries expanded rapidly.

Meat packing plants

The conditions at meat packing plants were good for the virus to spread. Large numbers of workers toil closely. Workers lift and manipulate heavy cuts of meat. Doing this requires breathing, which can transmit the virus to other workers. Some plants needed to provide masks, proper ventilation, or the means for adequate hygiene. With little or no testing, the virus could quickly spread before anyone noticed, and then it's too late. Eventually, some plants had to close after workers got sick and died. They had to clean the plant and provide protection to stop the spread of the virus.

Nursing home workers

The virus thrives in people with compromised health. Older adults with heart, lung, and circulation issues were quite vulnerable to the overpowering virus. In the beginning, workers didn't have masks and equipment to minimize the spread of the virus. Ventilation may not have been working or adequate to provide fresh air. In this context, many low-paid nursing home workers were quite vulnerable to the virus.

Transit workers

Large sectors of transport shut down. Commuter buses had less demand as people couldn't work in large offices, and city buses had fewer riders. Transit workers were laid off; some lost their jobs when commuter traffic took a nose dive.

Glut of jobs

I doubt anyone predicted a glut of jobs in the economy. Trump reduced the number of immigrants coming into the country. The Coronavirus killed many workers. With many workers saving money and not spending during the pandemic, they could choose whether or not to work. If the right job didn't come along, they could stay unemployed, which, for some, paid more than what they could make at a job. With more money in their pockets, people began spending as government restrictions on the economy faded. This led to an increase in demand for goods and services. The economy kept going strong. People wanted to buy houses and cars, but credit was expensive as the Fed raised interest rates to calm inflation.

Truckers

The trucking economy has been in flux. The pandemic is likely a speed bump in making trucks powered by batteries. The push to stop using fossil fuels to power trucks and automate them was in full swing before the pandemic. Some estimate that many trucking jobs will vanish within the next 15 years as electric AI-operated trucks do the job safer, faster, more efficient, and less expensive. This could still happen, but the opposite is also happening. Truckers are a critical link in the economy. The grocery shelves aren't stocked without them, and the money doesn't flow into corporate pockets. A shortage of truckers could destroy the economic output of many factories. It may take a significant amount of time to make the transition. Recently, Walmart announced it would pay nearly double the price for truckers. This may draw the best talent and signal to other companies that they must pay higher wages to get the job done as companies compete for labor. So, like many areas of the economy, the activity went way down during the pandemic and way up after, as pent-up demand and a surplus of spending money added fuel to a hot economy. As the supply of workers goes down, their wages increase. Years ago, Republican policies sought to increase the labor supply by letting immigrants into the country. Trump reversed that with a campaign against immigrants, who he scapegoated for many problems in the country, and used anger against immigrants as a way to get the white vote. At the same time, many small and large businesses hire immigrants because they work hard, pay the rent, and add color and culture to boring towns.

The great resignation

For some, it is no surprise that millions of workers would say no to endless toil for low pay. Some have worked for decades at low-paying jobs where incomes didn't keep up with inflation. They knew their money bought less, and the endless hours of dull, monotonous, and tedious work left their lives empty, hollow, and, for some, depressing and alienating. Those who didn't conform to the immediate dictates of the system would not be included in the benefits. Only some have the means or desire to attend college, join a union, or become a government employee. So, after the pandemic hit and the government began to pay decent unemployment, many workers realized that another life could be possible.

With time off and extra money, many have used the advantage of upgrading their housing. That backlog of building maintenance was about to shrink. Spending at home improvement stores soared. The extra time and money generated many home improvements. Other people took the time to develop hobbies or to check off items on their bucket list. With more time to draw, write, or make art, people realized that life wasn't only about work and making money.

Working from home was a significant improvement, which allowed more time, money, and energy for other things. Government payments made life easier and more secure.

Some people commute up to five hours a day. People who walk or bicycle may be exposed to traffic danger, accidents, pollution, construction fumes, and dust. These dangers may cause injury, death, and serious illnesses. They suffer the negative consequences of the vehicle users, which is quite unjust. The pandemic gave non-motorized commuters a break from the danger and injustice of the transport system, which favors motorized transport.

Frontline workers felt the most brutal blow from the pandemic; nurses, doctors, and hospital workers lost their lives and sanity as they faced an overwhelming stream of victims of the pandemic. Workers across the country and beyond lost their jobs. Restaurants, bars, theaters, and museum workers were hit hard. Many hardships could follow if you didn't have a job and didn't get unemployment or government assistance.

Chapter 13

Politics of action and inaction

What should the government do?

Take action or watch people die? If you had the lifeline, would you throw it away? For many in the US, the function of government is to facilitate exploitation, not to provide for the people's health, safety, and security.

Capitalism is driven to find the next big thing to turn pennies into gold. On the internet, it's your mind; in the grocery store, it's your stomach; in the hospital, it's your body. What will happen if you are not sick, hungry, and have books to read? There won't be any profits. A public health care system has an incentive to keep people healthy. If private health care aims to make money, capitalism is interested in making people sick, not healthy. If they are healthy, there's nothing to make money on. If the system prevents problems, profits will go down. If people use herbs that grow for free in wild areas around the house, their need to use the medical system may decrease. In the United States, the government's priority is to ensure that healthcare, education, and housing do not jeopardize profits.

Many people suffer and die from the virus as the Federal government fails to act.

The US had one of the highest death tolls from the virus. What does that say about the people in the country? The aging population in nursing homes was quite vulnerable to the virus. Is there ventilation and filtration of the air? If people eat low-nutrition, high-calorie foods that make them obese, what will happen? They get sick more frequently and die at a younger age than people who eat well and take care of themselves. Most stores are loaded with low-grade, heart disease, and cancer-causing foods that increase your chances of a visit to the hospital. Ever look at your hospital bills? Most who have done this realize what astronomical prices are standard. If you have insurance and don't have to pay, it's no big deal, or so people think. The United States spends the most on healthcare, while people get the least healthcare.

Thorough and rapid action by the Chinese government minimized the impact of the virus.

In China, the government took action to stop the virus. Instead of 1 million people dying, less than 10,000 died from the virus. Some say Chinese methods were too rough, too extreme, and overbearing. And what was done in the US? Trump destroyed the means to prevent a million people from dying from the virus. If you are a capitalist, why would you do things to make less money? capitalism makes the most money from people who are sick and dying.

Prevention

Prevention can prepare people to minimize the impact of the virus. G.W. Bush set up the means to do it when he was president. Since GW's time, all presidents, except Trump, have carried out the program, which set up testing, tracing, and isolating people to minimize the virus's spread. Governments that act in the public interest prevent problems before they start—not doing prevention before a pandemic is like living in a house without a roof during a hurricane. Suppose the government believes that corporations should profit from healthcare. In that case, the government has no interest in prevention; instead, it would dismantle prevention to increase profit, and that's what Trump did. Instead of the federal government negotiating to buy one large quantity for all, states were competing for personal protection equipment. Imagine welding without a helmet all day long. The lives of healthcare workers and hundreds of thousands of lives were fodder for the profiteering corporations. The more sick and dead, the more money they make. Now, if your priority is the health and safety of your people, you know that one ounce of prevention equals a pound of cure. With prevention, you get a massive bang for your buck. You won't have to stop bullets if no one has a gun. The government is not about prevention; if it were, all processed food would be taxed according to the health care consequences it generates.

Governor of New York, Andrew Cuomo, shut down the main functions of the economy to reduce the spread of the virus and preserve the function of the health care system. By the time the governor declared a state of emergency, the virus had spread to many areas of New York. After gutting the public hospitals, there was little space for patients. The for-profit hospitals operate at capacity or close to it. Excess, unused capacity is a drain on profits. With appropriate management, public hospitals could find a way to keep enough facilities open for a large-scale emergency. Perhaps it could be set up so people are on call for public service.

Chapter 14

Media

The pandemic spread fear, anxiety, and uncertainty in the public. News organizations were flooded with false information from the government, corporations, and others. With the facts and coherent information, the public could educate themselves about what should be done to protect the health and safety of family, friends, and neighbors. Corporations and governments competed for public support—the glut of information and competition for attention created confusion, uncertainty, and chaos.

The media reports what is fact and false; figuring out what is fact or fiction takes effort.

The media should report the positive things the government is doing.

The media reports critical ideas about the government's response.

The media should report how other countries have responded to the virus.

The media could report more of the scientific details of the virus.

The media should educate the public about solutions to current problems.

The news should focus on how people can stay safe, secure, and happy.

The news should report how our government, infrastructure, organization, and workers will help people through the pandemic with minimal consequences.

Some websites corroborate statements that appear to state facts.

How do we know that the fact-checking organizations are doing their job responsibly?

We can examine their sources and determine if they are reputable.

Do they have a history of lying?

What is their motivation for reporting?

What money will they gain if their stories are true?

Are there ways to corroborate what they say?

How can people corroborate facts?

Is the fact consistent with my experience?

Is the fact consistent with the experiences of people I know and trust?

Is the fact consistent with reputable information sources?

Does the source of the facts have a good track record of telling the truth?

Does the fact affect the reporter's influence, power, and monetary value?

Can the facts be measured?

How do these sources of facts make money?

What is at stake?

If the problem is overstated or understated, resources, time, energy, and money may be wasted, and people could suffer more pain, illness, and death.

Misinformation about the nature of the problem can restrict government action and prevent it from responding appropriately at the right time and place.

Echoing the lies

According to Trump and the Republican party, the pandemic was under control the whole time they were in office. Many reporters are trained not to question the words of the president. Anything the president says is news, even if it's a lie. For many in the media, it didn't matter if it was a lie. Lies make more money. What were the lies? Trump kept saying that the virus was going away and that fewer people were getting sick and dying when the opposite was the case. If the virus is going down, the government is doing the right thing and doesn't need to do anything else. The lies provided a cover for the failure of the government to protect people from the virus.

Trump lies

It's pretty astonishing how much a president can lie and never be held accountable, or the government has to make an extraordinary case to convict him because he has so many lawyers.

The following statements are lies:

Trump banned travel from China and Europe in time to prevent the spread of the virus.

At the beginning of the pandemic, the government provided personal protective equipment for frontline workers, and White House briefings informed the public about the virus.

The government did all it could to prevent the spread of the virus and to control the virus.

The election of 2020 was not legitimate and was stolen.

Reactive Media

In 2005, the government of George W. Bush made comprehensive plans to respond to a pandemic. The plan directed money to develop and stockpile vaccines and antiviral drugs, detect outbreaks, and prepare emergency plans. Solutions were known and in place, but Trump's government dismantled those plans and policies. As the pandemic raged, the Trump administration barely knew what to do. The media could have put more pressure on the government by educating the public about how to respond to the pandemic. It was up to the states to enact and carry out a plan to deal with the pandemic. The media should have informed the public how the government could respond in a coordinated national way to fight the virus. Without a coherent national plan, states would compete with other states for resources, equipment, and professionals like doctors and nurses. A proactive media would have outlined coherent national policies to respond to the virus. In the la la land of reaction and profits, the lives of many were put on the line as the president was out to lunch, watching TV, or playing golf.

Media bias

All media is biased. Some are biased by pretending to tell both sides of the story. You can hear the Democratic version or the Republican version; both versions are capitalism. The assumption is that there are two sides. There may be many other sides to the story that could be told. Usually, that is the case. So it's a matter of what is said and what is not. Stories focus on facts that support one side of the story. Most people experienced fear and anxiety during the pandemic. Some sought to deny what was happening, while others sought solutions.

Corporate media

Corporate media tells its story. What matters for a corporation? How it will make money is part of the equation. How will it affect the corporation's future profit potential?

The media should have informed the public about relevant and appropriate solutions for the government to explore. The press could have pressured the government to:

Provide protective equipment to frontline responders at the beginning of the pandemic.

Develop a coordinated national response to the pandemic to keep the economy moving without spreading the virus.

Put more emphasis on communicating what worked and what didn't work.

Reporting on the virus

We started hearing about the virus in China at the end of 2019. Many wanted to believe that the virus originated in China and spread throughout the rest of the world. Some sources say that the virus was in Europe in 2019. With little preparation, media outlets could not prepare the public for the pandemic. Worse yet, the government, under the guidance of Donald Trump, dismantled the government systems to deal with the pandemic.

Contradictions in the administration

With the president of the US lying daily, a large number of people began moving in the wrong direction. If you believe in a leader, you will do as they do. In this case, Trump refused to wear a mask, which may have led to many other people not wearing a mask and spreading the virus. Republicans had large gatherings where people did not wear masks. This violated social distancing rules and spread the virus far and wide.

Conspiracy theories multiplied, and extremists competed for territory, especially someone like Tucker Carlson. Doctor Fauci was in charge of the institutional government's response. Fauci told people to wear a mask and social distance, which is the opposite of what Trump was doing. This created even more conflict. The government was sending different messages. In the chaos of it all, 1 million people died while Trump and his buddies watched TV, played golf, and ate junk food. They were supposed to be stopping the virus from killing a million people.

Dominant media broadcasts lies from the administration.

How can a reporter respond to lies coming from those in the highest position of power? You must be courageous and able to take enormous risks, like losing your job, family, or life. It's a hazardous job, especially if you broadcast information that puts someone in jail, reduces their power, or puts a corrupt person in prison or reduces their power or profits. Some news organizations do this and get the rewards and suffer the consequences. The media is corporate in the United States and must make money. If an organization is low on cash or does not run well, it chooses what sells papers more than the facts and perspectives that would save a million people. Corrupt politicians threaten news organizations that undermine their power. Corroborated facts are the fundamental building blocks for reporters.

Lies and Consequences

What if the business leaders and reporters want to believe the lies? After all, who wants to deal with the painful news about a raging pandemic that is about to bring the country and your family and friends to their knees? It doesn't matter if you don't believe the government should care for its people. Remember that reporters who challenge what makes money end up dead in many places. Environmental reporters and human rights reporters go to war zones to liberate people from the oppressive conditions of the state. Would you put your life on the line to tell the facts as they are? What if you knew you would get fired? Many people wanted to believe the president. Am I willing to open my doors to a refugee, or a refugee from the injustice of the world, or my neighborhood, city, and nation? Someone said, "Speak truth to power," which sounds good, but are people adequately supported? A housing collective can produce high-quality, low-cost housing fueled by sweat equity and political participation to decide how to own, manage, and maintain your housing. Reporters with low-cost, decent housing will have energy for their jobs and lives and more integrity as they need less money.

Is "freedom of speech" more important than people's lives?

China shut down the virus by taking fast and thorough action, which didn't allow time for people to complain, and if people didn't comply with orders, they were forced to do it or be taken to prison. Is it more important for people to be able to speak their minds or more essential to stop the virus from taking people's lives? With all the mind garbage and brainwashing of the public and grandiose platitudes, it makes sense to have people comply with a few rules to save the lives of many. Is freedom of speech worth a million lives? Is it OK to be quiet and listen?

Chapter 15

Political Economy

Large sectors of the economy shut down. Many workers were laid off. Initially, the federal government stopped the government from cooperating to provide safety equipment and tests for the virus and educate people about the importance of acting in a unified way to stop the virus. The virus spread quickly. People didn't know what was going on. Believe the lies or believe your eyes. We were told to wash hands frequently, avoid getting within 6 feet of someone, and to wear a mask outside the house. If you stayed away from the virus until the vaccine was available, you could avoid dying. Some groups were hit hard by the virus, and others had incomes to cushion them from the virus.

Trump's response to the pandemic

Trump dismantled the pandemic response administration and workforce shortly after taking office. Previous presidents, both Republican and Democratic, had set up a pandemic response plan and prepared the government to respond. Plans were implemented to ensure emergency responders had personal protection equipment. Trump stopped government workers from responding appropriately to the pandemic. Hundreds of thousands of people likely died from that decision. If Trump had done nothing, many in government would have taken action and prevented many from the fate of the virus. Trump was against the Centers for Disease Control.

The government had to educate the public or communicate in some way. In dire straits without enough equipment, hospital staff, workers, nurses, and doctors complained that they had to work without proper safety equipment. This put them and their patients in harm's way. If many doctors and nurses were ill or dead, the ability of society to minimize the impact of the virus would be hampered at best. Forward-looking public officials saw it coming and took action to provide equipment, resources, and directions. Suddenly, in part, because the federal government didn't buy in bulk, states competed for life-saving supplies, equipment, and machines.

The government expands payments to workers.

Pandemic Unemployment Assistance paid workers directly. Sometimes, these payments were as much as or more than income from their jobs, providing an incentive not to work. Without a break for many years, people began to realize what life could be without the constant emergency of getting to and from work, fixing and parking the car, and running endlessly to chase a life of consumption and production. Many had no idea what life could be without the eternal treadmill of the rat race.

Governments enforce eviction moratoriums.

Governments enacted an eviction moratorium to prevent the spread of the virus. The law was supposed to prevent people from moving from one house or apartment to another. Tenants invited other people to live with them during the pandemic. The law prevented landlords from getting paid rent. Some people moved into occupied apartments and turned the apartments into shooting galleries, brothels, and houses for criminals. They destroyed the rental units. The government took control of the buildings and let the tenants live for free, destroy the building, and make a nuisance. With no laws to prevent people from moving into occupied apartments, the laws failed to prevent people from moving into apartments and spreading the virus. So, tenants were protected from government eviction. The government decides whether or not a tenant is evicted. Only the government can evict a tenant. The government stopped evicting tenants during the moratorium. The government's eviction program is a substitute for housing. Instead of making housing, the government evicts people.

Labor Supply problems

After the government shut down nonessential sectors of the economy, demand for goods and services decreased. Businesses didn't need alcohol for bars, food and equipment for restaurants, and gas for buses. As the people developed immunity to the virus, the government started to open up the economy. With pockets full of money from the pandemic payments, people were ready to spend. Pent-up demand and a shortage of workers set up the conditions for workers to demand higher pay. Unions and the condition for wage increases arrived. With many workers dead from the virus, fewer immigrants, and a swelling demand for homes, cars, and consumer goods, labor would be in short supply. The capitalist project is now pushing harder and faster to run the planet into extinction. Fetishistic consumption doesn't help people. The push to make billions of consumers generate vast amounts of waste will run the planet into extinction.

Were the Chinese doing a better job protecting their people from the virus?

Compared to the US, China's ability to build a hospital or test millions in one city in less than ten days was an achievement most Western countries could only dream of. As of June 2022, less than 7,000 Chinese died from the virus. They knew how to contain and prevent the virus from getting from city to city. This is a stunning achievement. Perhaps the country has a more homogenous population that is more willing to follow orders or identify with the needs of the country and do what is needed to defeat the virus, even if it means staying home for three months without working. If your needs are met, is that such a bad deal? A public health care system works to prevent and minimize health problems by prioritizing prevention. You save many times if you put a significant effort into stopping the virus before it can get going. An ounce of prevention is worth a pound of cure. In the West, you can make more money on a pound of cure, and in the US, thinking about what is good for the group is a foreign idea to most. The Chinese have mastered the art of cooperation and unification for everyone's interest. Of course, many may disagree and get the short end of the stick, but in the long term, the Chinese protected their citizens from the main impact of the virus. Are the Chinese more for freedom than the US? If you are dead, can you be free? A few may say yes, but most would rather be alive. Were there some people who didn't want to comply and were roughed up by the authorities? This could be the case, and then again, are you better off being roughed up or dead from a pandemic that the government failed to stop?

The Chinese response to the virus.

It seems evident that the Chinese response to the pandemic was done well, especially compared to the United States. The number of dead is a stunning fact; in China, less than 7,000 people died from the virus. In the US, over 1 million people died. Yes, China has used some authoritarian methods to make people comply, but those people are alive now. In the US, most would be dead.

Chapter 16

Nonhuman entities

As the economic shock spread and many businesses, schools, and activities shut down, the assault on the natural world subsided. With fewer businesses open and fewer people traveling, animals were less likely to get killed crossing highways and were less afraid to explore urban areas with fewer people. Animals roamed into parks, cities, and urban landscapes. More birds made the skies come alive. Another world actualized in the difference,

The big silence opening

The roar of the city stopped. A garbage truck, ambulance, fire truck, loud music, or something sounds off frequently in NYC. As the urban cacophony subsides, areas for the birds to sing, dogs to bark, and fairies to bring the magic of life opened up. The big machine became still, and the city transformed into a peaceful, sleepy Sunday afternoon that makes you wish it would last forever. The tranquility of the environment was a stark contrast to the usual hustle and bustle, offering a moment of calm in the chaos.

Liberation from the fossil fuel economy

The economic slowdown meant fewer vehicles would pollute the air, land, and water. Not much was mentioned in the news, but people who ride a bicycle or walk could smell and taste the difference. Without a barrage of smoke, dust, and pollution, people had fewer headaches, respiratory issues, and stress as people stopped driving. Those with lung issues got a hiatus from the assault, which appears ordinary but is deadly.

Chapter 17

Disorientation

The pandemic took people by surprise. This entity ambushed humans. All the armies of the world couldn't do what the virus did. Suddenly, it spread worldwide without shipping, the internet, or fossil fuels. Invisible, everywhere, and more deadly than the most enormous army, how could this happen? Bewildered, people kept going.

Once every hundred years

After the 9/11 terrorist attacks, I got this feeling like I and the world were at a turning point. Things will never be the same. Something big would be different, and I didn't know what it was. When the virus hit, and the server told me they would be closed indefinitely, it felt like a mega-shift. Both events were once-in-a-lifetime events. While the two events aren't comparable in scale, both events overturned assumptions about our world. Few would imagine the airplanes flying into the World Trade Center on a suicide mission. The pandemic was similar. People could not imagine what an intense and profound impact it would have.

Anti-social disorientation in low-density US

I came to NYC to escape the low-density US. Except for small inner city areas, most of the urban landscape is dominated by residential neighborhoods where few people walk the streets. It's like a neutron bomb wiped out all the people. The assumption is that people want to own a car and a wife, go to Church, eat white bread, and guard their backyard. Furthermore, people shouldn't use a public park; transit is inconvenient, low class, and too dangerous for white, middle-class people, and you should be afraid of and not talk to anyone who isn't as white as the bread. Outside of some areas in LA, San Francisco, Chicago, and New York City, most other urban areas have small pockets of human activity at best. Social activity is mostly permitted in shopping malls, churches, and military parades. If you don't own a car, go to Church, or go shopping, you are abnormal and belong in an institution.

Anxiety

The pandemic fueled an epidemic of anxiety as people witnessed their lives torn apart. The slow onslaught of the viral death machine circulated an ominous future; who would be alive in 6 months or 12 months? What family and friends would the virus kill? If you didn't live with a close group of friends or family, you might not have anyone to help you recover from the virus, or, in isolation, you could get lonely and, worse, depressed. Many lost their jobs overnight. Imagine that I have no job, and the virus is about to kill me or my family or friends.

Numerous fears crumbled the security of the pre-pandemic era. As that security, the social glue from interactions at school, work, shopping, or casual strolls through the park vanished, a subtle disorientation enveloped the nation. To the extent that social culture vanished, to that extent, anxiety and depression spread. People with money in the bank, a house in the countryside, and family or friends at home had the advantage. Also, if you had a therapist, you had another advantage. The great majority felt their world disintegrating.

Depression

If you were lonely or had a lot of negative thoughts and tendencies before the pandemic, the onset of the virus could make you closer to a severe illness. Losing a friend or loved one, seeing them in pain, or getting a severe case of the virus could make the depression worse. Many lost their job and income without any warning. Others feared the virus so much they didn't leave the house for months. Getting over that may take a lot of time or some good LSD.

Fear in the pandemic

The lack of government and media preparation to educate the public about the pandemic caused many problems. People needed to figure out what to do or what to expect. People didn't know how to respond to the virus. The government told us what to do. We had to stay home and only go out if we had a mask and gloves on. We could go to the grocery store, pharmacy, and maybe a hospital. That bedrock institution, the hospital, was now thrown into jeopardy by the virus. No one knew how long it would take before a vaccine was ready. Many people questioned whether a mask or social distancing effectively reduced the spread of the virus. Some had little to fear. If you lived below your means, you had enough money and knew how to live without undermining your future, even if it meant living without an income for a couple of years. Others living paycheck to paycheck were in dire straits. If you were vulnerable to the virus, you had much to fear. Before the vaccine was available, many wondered whether they would leave the hospital alive. Some assumed that if you get dropped off at the hospital with a severe Covid 19 illness, there was a good chance you'd never come out again.

Child anxiety and depression during the pandemic

Children suffered enormously during the pandemic. Even if their household was intact and they had the technology to go to school, the structure of their world fell apart. Many were swamped with too much activity and insufficient play and time with friends and fellow students. Some had friends in the neighborhood, but during COVID, the risk of spreading the virus limited how much time parents would allow children to be with their friends. People had little information about how to minimize or control it. We were told to wash our hands, wear masks, and practice social distancing. It wasn't clear how the virus was spread. Was it from droplets from the nose and mouth? Another idea is that it is like a cloud of smoke from your lungs, small particles that can easily float. That's what they said at the beginning of the pandemic. Anxiety and depression consumed many children. Some children lost connection with their parents and began using drugs to curb the pain. Unless the child interacted with a good therapist or had ample social activity, their world could slide downhill quickly.

They are spreading the virus without knowing it.

Schools, businesses, and government operations closed after the pandemic started. Somehow, society had to learn to live with the deadly virus. People on the front lines and people with jobs that exposed them to many people were quite vulnerable. The virus took hold before people were aware of it. People were infecting each other on a mass scale without any idea what was happening. Workers in restaurants, bars, grocery stores, school bus drivers, and security personnel may spread the virus without knowing it. Eventually, it became apparent that there was a difference between small and large amounts of exposure. If you were a person who only interacted with a few people or not very often, your risk was less.

Economic Shock

Many lost their jobs overnight. If you lived from paycheck to paycheck, your stress rose quickly. How could you work if the government shut down your employer? While the government provided money during the pandemic, those who were undocumented didn't qualify and faced an enormous struggle to survive. Even those with unemployment compensation were still determining if they would be employed again.

Emptiness in the city that never sleeps

In March 2020, Cuomo, the governor of New York state, shut down most activities. The virus had spread and was rapidly infecting and killing large numbers of people. It was too late to prevent the initial surge, but they did it anyway. Immediately, the number of people and vehicles in public plummeted. The streets were empty. Human activity vanished instantly. This invisible particle stopped cars and people immediately. Nothing else could do that, not even warfare. How could something be so invincible? It's a virus; it hit the jackpot of human weakness. What does the virus gain? Who, what, where, how, and why is its reason to exist? Perhaps the last time the streets were this empty was in the previous pandemic in 1918, one hundred years earlier. Numb and stunned, people kept going.

Abolition of desire

Many people flock to NYC for social action. Life is living in museums, theaters, bars, and restaurants. Without the pulse and energy on the street, what good is NYC? Yes, people come to see the built landscape of the urban arena, but it's more about the people. You see more difference in a few minutes on one corner than in most areas of the country. For NYC commuters, tourists, and citizens, the pandemic was like social solitary confinement that deadened the motivation to live to the fullest, engage in difference, and explore the range of options only available in NYC. Confused about how to live, disrupted by economic and social events, and unable to clarify their future, many needed guidance about their next moves. Without work, was it time to leave the city? Without culture and art, what was the point of life? When would the pandemic end and people finally be able to experience a life worth living?

Production of disorientation

It's common to see one or more people screened into their phones in public places and around the house chasing Artificial Intelligence (AI). For parents, children watching endless videos and consuming social media is an epidemic. The children don't get outside, exercise, engage in hobbies, or do their chores around the house. Some may have used this media as one of the last ways to stay with something that hasn't changed and something they can control. It's the ultimate power, freedom, and control. I get what I want instantaneously; now that's the spoiled American appetite, the ultimate seduction of the AI machine. Dealing with reality becomes the ultimate stretch and disorientation. Direct, unmediated experience may be impossible in the land of disorientation. With a cancer-like grip, it seizes the most precious gift of life, attention, and extracts enough bits of attention to make a sale. They need to get social food to feed their souls. AI is stealing the inner core of the child. Most public activity stopped after March 2020. Is radical subjectivity impossible in screen land?

Police murders during the pandemic destabilize security and justice.

The pandemic occurred while Trump was president. His policies and actions favored whites over everyone else. The assumption for many white people was that the white man was finally vindicated after years of being blamed for the problems of society. As this was happening, many whites in positions of power may have felt it was time to assert their privilege and put people in their place. After a white police officer in Minneapolis, Derek Chauvin murdered George Floyd, people around the country protested. People could not tolerate the senseless use of force while wearing a badge. Seeing the image of a black man dying as police officers and onlookers did nothing to stop it was disempowering and shocking. If you're not a white person, is it safe to go outside? Will the police come and kill me for doing nothing? If the police do arrive, should we watch and let them do what they do? or do we take action to prevent another senseless loss of life? Trying to stop the police is very dangerous and could result in them killing you. Videotaping events of the police using force could save lives, but police attack reporters. The shocking display of police brutality and abuse sparked a national response. For many, the whole experience; the trauma of seeing someone lose their life while others watch and do nothing, demands for change resulted in few if any gains, and the frequent mass shootings were enough to spin people out of it, to bring on a numbness to the assault on the peace and security of the neighborhood.

Chapter 18

Transition to a post-pandemic economy

Eventually, more people developed immunity after getting sick or getting the vaccine. The majority had an immune system that could prevent the virus from making them seriously ill or killing them. The virus did not threaten the healthcare system or the economy. Frontline workers could grab a sigh of relief. As the ordeal faded, people on the front lines transitioned to a more stable, secure future. Bars, restaurants, and hotels started to see customers come back. Employers with commuters began the uphill battle to get workers to start commuting.

Transport

Commuters resisted going back to pre-pandemic transportation the most. Commuting is a waste of time, energy, and money. People who drive could get tickets, be stranded on the highway because the car broke down, or get stuck in bad weather or an accident. Working from home meant they would have more time with family, more time to do non-work activities and save time, energy, and money. Some refused to return to work and lost their jobs, a few moved closer to work, and many started commuting again. Transit was slow to move to pre-pandemic levels. Eager to get back in action and bridled by the government's requirement to keep the venues safe, bars, restaurants, and entertainment venues gradually open their doors. Without buses and trains bringing in loads of commuters, the businesses had to adjust to the grueling conditions of post-pandemic America.

Housing

After the eviction moratorium ended, the government began evicting people in January 2022 in New York State. Many landlords needed help to pay for housing. Many tenants owed five or even $10,000 or more. Although ERAP paid for some housing, many tenants did not pay during the pandemic, which was very costly for the landlords. Because the laws had changed, it needed to be clarified to many tenants and landlords what the law was. Often, the laws have language that must be interpreted by a lawyer or judge specializing in landlord-tenant law. I've been in court when the judge or lawyers ask each other what the law is, and they try to figure it out. At the end of the pandemic, many tenants were not paying rent. Many had money but knew the courts would not push them to pay. If judges are elected, they may get more votes if they favor the tenant. In New York State, most of the government favors the tenant. New York State needs to produce more affordable housing. There are many laws that the landlord must comply with, and tenants who pay rent have to pay the bill for tenants who don't pay rent. Also, it's nearly impossible for a landlord to hold the tenant accountable for destroying the property or disturbing the peace.

The landlord must prove beyond a reasonable doubt to the judge that the tenant is violating the lease. This requires enormous time, energy, and money to pay lawyers and to pay for the apartment when the tenant stops paying. While this is happening, the tenant-landlord relationship deteriorates. Many tenants know the process. They know how to game the system. With the judges on their side and free lawyers, they can stay in the rental unit for months or years without paying rent. The government evicts tenants after allowing them to stay for months without paying. That way, the tenants will feel like they have won the game. Favoring the tenant will ensure more votes when the judge runs for office.

Condition of housing

The government took over housing. The government forced landlords to provide housing for free. During this time, the power was transferred from the landlord to the tenant and the government. The government dictated the conditions under which a landlord would get paid, and the landlord would only get paid if the tenant and landlord filled out all the paperwork correctly for ERAP. For many tenants, it didn't matter if they filled out the paperwork; they knew that the government would never make them pay for housing in New York State. So, delinquent tenants had little incentive to enroll in the ERAP program. When tenants know they don't have to pay, they feel the power. Some use this as a green light to destroy the apartment. When the tenant goes to court and shows photos of a busted-up and damaged apartment, the judge will quickly determine that they do not have to pay rent because the apartment is damaged. Also, the tenant can call the building department, and the building department will issue a violation to the landlord.

The landlord will be required to fix what the tenant destroys. Many of these tenants will not let the landlord in to correct the problem. This increases the tension. So, given all these conditions, housing deteriorated during the pandemic. This is another factor that led to the increase in housing prices. The government made it very hard for a landlord to petition the government to evict the tenant. What does that mean? The landlord must pay more time, energy, and money to evict the tenant, meaning they must increase the rent. Again, the tenants who pay end up paying for those who don't. The government tells tenants that they don't have to pay, can destroy the housing, and can bother anyone at any time unless the landlord proves to the judge that the tenant is breaking the lease. The government makes it extremely difficult for a landlord to prove that the tenant is not paying, breaking things, or bothering people. All of this drives up the cost of housing. The government wants affordable housing and is doing many things to make sure housing is unaffordable. During the pandemic, many housing units were destroyed or damaged because of the government policies. This drives up rent.

Economy

The government paid unemployed workers, people who suffered economic damage during the pandemic, and businesses to keep them operating. Some of these were generous payments for people who manage their money well. They used this money to pay for expenses and renovations and save money. Eventually, employers called people back to work. Some people didn't want to commute and quit their jobs. Other people realized that low-income work could not provide a life worth living. Large numbers stopped working. They lived on what savings they had, lived with their parents, or became homeless. Some of them found jobs that were closer to home and paid more money. Because many people died and many refused to go back to work, the labor pool shrank and businesses struggled to find workers. Immigrants saw the green light and provided fresh energy to the dwindling workforce. Wages and unions began to increase. Inflation began to spiral after the government gave a lot of money to workers and businesses.

Education

During the pandemic, students had to take classes from home using their computer with an Internet connection. This led to many problems but kept the system going. People require social interaction to be healthy. Many children did not get this during the pandemic—this led to an epidemic of mental health issues, including anxiety and depression. Schools had to make sure the students were safe. Schools require vaccination of students, staff, and teachers. Some people resisted and could not get into school. Opening the schools generated significant conflict between those who wanted to wait and those who wanted it open. Some said the schools were unsafe, and most wanted the children to return to in-school learning, where children could socialize, make friends, and learn something. Most agreed that students learn more in person at school and that schools should be open as soon as possible. In New York City, schools did online classes from March 2022 to September 2023.

Healthcare system

The pandemic tested the healthcare system. Quickly, the pandemic overwhelmed the healthcare system of New York City as a massive surge of COVID-19 patients needed care. With little or no experience with this virus and a pandemic, nurses and doctors scrambled to help patients. Without a good solution at hand, healthcare professionals did the best they could. Twenty thousand people died in the first three months when the pandemic hit New York City. Noncritical health care was delayed or canceled.

The pandemic challenged governments, businesses, and people to adapt to the dangers of the virus. In China, the communist party responded quickly, making the virus impossible to spread. Just before the pandemic hit the United States, Donald Trump, President at the time, dismantled the government that was prepared to respond to a pandemic. Trump's goal was to increase profits for corporations. As the pandemic quickly killed 20,000 New Yorkers in months, the president was forced to admit there was a big problem. The government's failure especially hit frontline workers, older people, and youth. Eventually, the death toll would rise to over 1 million people as it became apparent that the priority of the government was profits more than people.

About the Author

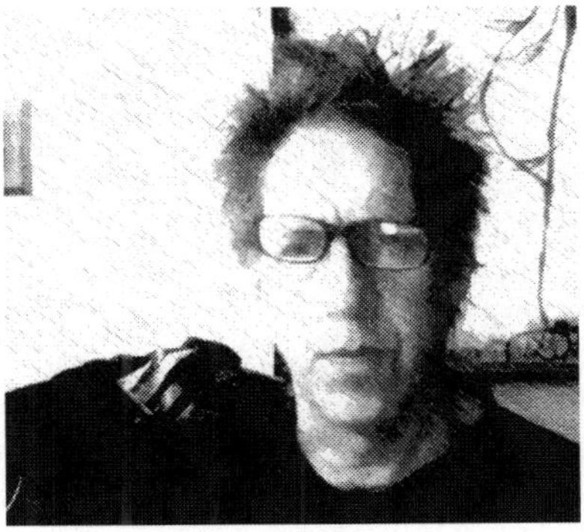

Dan Paul grew up in Lake Wobegon fishing, playing sports and building houses. After attending the University of Wisconsin, Madison and working at the linear fusion reactor lab, he explored alternatives to the dominant codes. While staying in coops, communes, and squats around the country, he learned the fundamentals of setting up and operating progressive, radical and sustainable alternatives to the code of the corporation and nation.

Also by Dan Paul

Philosophy of Action Design and Multiplicity by Dan Paul

Book 1 Auto Free Design

Book 2 Workers Health Handbook

Book 3 Save Your Life Prevent Hospital Use

Book 4 Coop Owners Handbook

Book 5 Eye on AI Meeting Needs Sustainably

Book 6 Travels on the Nomadic Terrain

Book 7 Tales of the Urban Shaman

Book 8 Housing in the Danger Zone

Book 9 Corona Time

Book 10 Philosophy of Design, Action and Multiplicity

Coming soon

Landlords Against Eviction

Auto Free USA

Websites

https://viaradmedia.org

https://autofreedesign.com

http://workershealthhandbook.com

http://sylphu.com

Made in the USA
Monee, IL
09 November 2026

67380384R00073